Praise for

AFTER SHOCK: From Cancer Diagnosis to Healing

"**... a much needed and valuable guide to support anyone entering the world of cancer** diagnosis and treatment, be it traditional, complementary, or a well researched and thought-through combination of the two. **Highly recommended for patients, family, friends and caregivers...**"

Joyce Goodrich, Ph.D., Past President, Consciousness Research and Training Project, Inc. (Lawrence LeShan approach to healing) 1929-2009

"I highly recommend the insights and practical value of this balanced and compassionate book for anyone facing cancer. It is **an important tool of personal empowerment** at a time when so many people feel that their life is beyond their control."

June Peoples-Mallon, Long-time Executive Producer of the national public radio program "The Infinite Mind"

"**... a practical, wise companion to those facing cancer.** Puja Thomson's insightful guidance and holistic approach helps patients lighten the burden of a diagnosis, clarify options and reveals how a cancer experience can become a pilgrimage for healing."

Janet Hand, MA, RN, founder of Pathways to Wellness Healing Center and former faculty at Adelphi University School of Nursing

"Puja has given us **an operating manual, not only to survive cancer, but also to grow through it.** It is a caring and knowledgeable compendium to have with you in the difficult transition from diagnosis through treatment. I couldn't put the book down. I encourage you to go out and read this if you have cancer or know anyone who does."

Jason Elias, MA, LAc, Author of *Feminine Healing* and *Chinese Medicine for Maximum Immunity*

"A personal perspective, such as Ms. Thomson's, is so **very importan**
decisions about healing."
Ann Fonfa, President, The Annie Apple!

"**...the best bottom line, down-to-earth, easy reading and mo book** I have ever read on the subject... No one diagnosed should be book."

Gina C., Pennsylvania Breast Cancer Coalit

"*AFTER SHOCK*... is practical, easy to follow and **very comprehen!** needs to be in the offices of every health care professional from (nurses to therapists and pharmacies."

Rosalyn Cherry LMT, Patient and Massage Therapist

Special Edition/Third Printing 2008
Revised Edition Copyright © 2016

1. Cancer 2. Health 3. Self-help 4. Body, Mind and Spirit
ISBN 978-1-928663-09-6
Library of Congress Control Number 2015948566

Published by ROOTS & WINGS, New Paltz, NY. Printed in the USA
Design: Tory Ettlinger
Logo: Helene Sarkis   Cover art: Samantha Thomaier with Christian Zeiler

*Grateful acknowledgement is made to the following sources
for permission to reprint copyrighted material:*

Osho International Foundation for quote from *Osho Transformation Tarot* by Osho © Osho International Foundation Switzerland. www.osho.com: reprinted with permission.

Nancy Wood for her poems *My Help is in the Mountain* from *Spirit Walker* © Nancy Wood, Delacorte 1993 and *Earth Cure Me* from *Hollering Sun* © Nancy Wood, Simon and Schuster 1973, both used by permission.

Marion Woodman for excerpts from *BONE: Dying into Life* © Marion Woodman: reprinted with permission.

Dr. Valerie Hunt for the quote from *Infinite Mind* © Dr Valerie Hunt, Malibu Press: reprinted with permission.

Quotes from Dr. Barrie Cassileth are also included with permission.

Please note: This book is designed with the understanding that the author and publisher are not engaged in rendering individualized professional services. The suggestions, explorations and questions are intended for individual and group study and are not designed to be a substitute for professional consultation. Furthermore, vignettes are intended to illustrate the varied challenges, issues and choices facing cancer patients. They do not imply endorsement of any specific treatment by the author or publisher.

Address all inquiries to:

Roots & Wings
PO Box 1081
New Paltz, NY 12561

info@rootsnwings.com
www.rootsnwings.com/aftershock

AFTER SHOCK:
FROM CANCER DIAGNOSIS TO HEALING

A step-by-step guide to navigate your way

Puja A. J. Thomson

ROOTS & WINGS PUBLISHING
New Paltz, New York

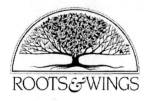

ROOTS&WINGS

—

Dedication

It is with great love and respect that I dedicate this book in honor of four remarkable people and their courageous journeys.

Two, whose youthful physical lives were snuffed out prematurely by cancer, but who both live on through the inspiration and immense courage they manifested throughout their cancer experiences. It was a privilege to be touched by their irrepressible spirits:

JEREMY CAHILL
Jeremy, the jaunty angle of your baseball hat said it all.

KATIE SCHOLL
*Katie, your smile is in the gold and brown sunflowers
you loved so much.*

And two beloved friends whose experience with cancer
came later in life:

MATTHEW FASOLINO
*Matthew, your indomitable spirit, on and off the tennis court, enriched
my life. You created new spaces in my home from the sauna to the loft
and your nourishing meals—buckwheat blueberry pancakes, escarole and
beans—sustained me through hours of writing.*

JANE FERBER, M.D.
*Jane, you opened your home and heart to me at a challenging time in my
life. Your silver Maine-blueberry pendant necklace, a gift to your healing
team, continues to remind me of the great natural circle of life.*

This revised edition is dedicated
to the many cancer patients who face daily challenges with courage
and faith and who continue to inspire me.

—

Contents

Reach In—Create Your Own Wellness Program

Moving Forward

Acknowledgements

I HAVE BEEN EXCEEDINGLY BLESSED IN THE GENEROUS, OPEN-hearted help I have received from many people throughout the writing of this book:

Special and profound thanks to Barbara Sarah, Founder of the Oncology Support Program at HealthAlliance Hospital in Kingston, NY, who first planted the seed and then nurtured its growth with her constant support and lively spirit. She used her amazing networking skills to facilitate connections to many others on my behalf.

From start to finish, Alice Goodman generously offered her medical writing and editorial skills. My writing buddies, Miki Frank and Joyce Reeves, helped me express my voice over numerous cups of tea. Alice, Miki and Joyce were unstinting in their encouragement from their different perspectives. Their constructive criticism, spiked with good humor and laughter, contributed immeasurably to greater clarity and many an enjoyable moment.

Others, including Donald Sarvananda Bluestone PhD, Kerry Cronin MD, Martha Elder, Sandra Fisher, Kathleen Folliard RN, Joyce Goodrich PhD, Janet Hand MA RN, Patrice Heber, Beth Stewart and Elizabeth Tapen MD, contributed suggestions at early phases of writing or to different aspects of the content, while Sheldon Feldman MD FACS,

Judith Roth DC, and Melissa Wood reviewed and helped me fine-tune the book.

I didn't have to look very far for vignettes to illustrate challenges and choices. I was deeply touched that, without hesitation, Donald Sarvananda Bluestone, Joan Casamo, Linda Clarke, Mary Cropper, Diana Edelman, Tory Ettlinger, Esther Frances, Jan Guthrie, Marty Laforse, Lilly Mathisen, Kathleen McBride, Miriam Patton, Ujjala Schwartz, Phyllis Sturm, Tona Wilson, Melissa Wood and Marion Woodman (and others who wish to remain anonymous) were so willing to pass on what they had learned from their experience.

My gratitude also goes to Tory Ettlinger for the lay-out design, a work of art and a labor of love that without a doubt exquisitely supports the intention of the text; Ginger Graziano for the evocative cover of the original edition, Samantha Thomaier and Christian Zeiler for the hopeful cover of the revised edition; and to all those who have helped in other ways—Perri Ardman, Joan Casamo, Anthony Clark, Linda Clarke, Brigit Fasolino-Vucic, David and Susan Jamon, Megan Joiner, Angelika Leik, Erica Manfred, Hope Nemiroff, Diana Waldron and my twin brother Iain M. Thomson. I am also appreciative of many other conversations and emails—too numerous to mention.

I wish to express my heartfelt appreciation for the practical, emotional and spiritual help I received during the intensity of my personal cancer pilgrimage over twelve years ago: profound thanks to friends who accompanied me to medical appointments and took time to prepare and review the visits, exploring endless questions with me; to all who contributed their professional expertise, both mainstream and complementary and for all the sustenance through prayer and healing energy from my family and many friends near and far, especially my long-time hands-on-healing circle.

Lastly, many thanks to the patients, family members and others who took the time to encourage me, by calling or writing to share how *After Shock:*... had eased their journey since the first edition.

I have been fortunate indeed. Thank you, one and all.

Foreword

OH, HOW I WISH THAT I HAD THE BOOK YOU ARE ABOUT to read when I was initially diagnosed with breast cancer in April of 1992! I remember sitting in the doctor's office across the desk from him while he spoke to me about my treatment options, outcomes and statistics. I have this visceral image of myself, nodding in agreement, while the words floated over my head. It was as if a glass window had come down between us; I could see my doctor talking but couldn't hear the words. Thanks to cancer, I decided to become an oncology social worker so that I could accompany patients to their appointments to be a second pair of ears; someone who could ask questions, take notes and offer support. When the meeting was over, I could process the session with the patient, clarify the information that had been given and offer to assist if further research was required.

Fast forward eleven years to December 2003—I had been accompanying patients to their medical appointments for ten years and knew personally and professionally a great deal about the stress and anxiety they undergo. As I was sitting with Puja Thomson waiting for her appointment with her surgeon, we began to review her questions and concerns.

She then wrote down some notes in her loose-leaf binder. I asked to look at her book and she showed me how she had begun to organize all of the aspects of her cancer experience.

Now, I've always advised patients to keep a book where they could write down their questions, reflections, information, resources, thoughts and feelings. Yet what Puja had organized was far beyond anything I had seen even though I had had the opportunity to review a great deal of published material collected by our Oncology Support Program. It was amazingly comprehensive. I immediately asked her if she would be willing to develop what she had structured for herself into a book, which I knew would be of great benefit to newly diagnosed cancer patients.

Here it is…all in one volume, beautifully written and organized, guiding you on your inner and outer journeys as you make choices of doctor and treatments, mainstream and complementary medicine, and deal with the many practical matters, questions and feelings that can easily overwhelm you. Puja's personal experience with breast cancer and her professional training and experience as an interfaith minister, creator of rituals, massage therapist, and Scottish organizer is a perfect combination to make the material that you are about to use the best possible method for organizing your cancer experience. We've gotten a lot of wonderful advice in the development of this project and I've been happy to encourage its unfolding. I believe that *After Shock: From Cancer Diagnosis to Healing*, thanks to Puja Thomson's talent and skill, continues to be unparalleled material for the successful navigation of anyone who wants to reduce the stress of their cancer journey. It will undoubtedly guide you step-by-step as you find your own way to recovery.

Barbara Sarah, LCSW
Founder of the Oncology Support Program
at HealthAlliance of the Hudson Valley, Kingston, New York.
Recipient of the 2005 New York State Governor's Award for
Innovation and Research in Breast Cancer.
Cancer Consultant, www.thirdopinion.net.
Fall 2015

Introduction

WHEN THE NEWS THAT I HAD CANCER EVENTUALLY PEN-
etrated my being in the doctor's office, I felt very
shaky. Caught off guard, I was surprised at how vulnerable
I had suddenly become. Nothing—not my competence as a
health practitioner, nor knowledge of cancer, nor experiencing the personal pain of an intimate friend's struggle to beat
"it" during the previous two years—nothing—prepared me
to face the verdict of cancer in my own body.

Pressured to make a quick decision about treatment, I felt
as if I was being sucked into a big machine and onto a con-
veyor belt. My doctor seemed to know exactly what I should
do before I even had a chance to get my bearings. Weighed
down by these demands and decisions, I took time to walk,
to meditate, and then share my news with a very few close
friends.

I realized I faced three challenges: I needed to ask for support from others, to find a way to bring clarity and order into
this fearful, confusing experience and to tap into my own
intuitive understanding. Along the way, as I acted in accordance with these awarenesses, I discovered precious gifts in
addition to those offered by my health practitioners. In asking
for what I wanted from others, my heart opened to the generosity of friends; I found that good organization lessened my

scattered energy; and in listening to myself, I began to allow a new balance to come into my life.

After Shock: From Cancer Diagnosis to Healing evolved out of my attempts to create a container and structure that would support my journey. From my first fledgling notes grew this tool to assist you in organizing your cancer experience, especially during the first crucial year. If you are facing an unwelcome recurrence, I hope you too will find this book helpful and encouraging. Its purpose is not to give detailed medical information or advice. I call on my personal and professional experience and training to offer practical suggestions and guidelines to help you clarify your own process, perspectives and choices. Woven throughout are stories shared by friends and fellow travelers as well as my own.

Reach Out

With the discovery of cancer, it's really helpful to ask for support from trusted friends and family. It's advisable to find out as much as you can about your type of cancer from sources such as your local library, cancer resource organizations and the Internet. Your life will shift, as mine did, to include an all-absorbing round of medical visits. As you search for the best possible professional care, you'll probably meet with your primary physician, surgeon and oncologist. Next come tests and treatment, waiting for and receiving results. Perhaps you'll get a second or third opinion, or seek out a complementary practitioner. You will make decision after decision about your treatment and deal with all sorts of medical records, financial statements, bills and insurance plans. At times such tasks may seem endless.

Get Organized

Disorganization is definitely hazardous to your health! I quickly discovered that good record keeping was essential if I were to avoid ending up under a mountain of paperwork. I was amazed at how quickly papers accumulated—personal jottings of conversations or dreams, medical prescriptions, exam results, bills and so on. In the early days I just lumped everything together and I dissipated precious energy by scrambling around to find a crucial piece of information from a pile of haphazard notes. Sorting things out is in fact a way of controlling this "runaway train." It will save lots of time and contribute to your sanity.

REACH IN

In the midst of all this hard work, I felt pulled in another direction. While first and foremost I wanted to heal my physical body, I knew that more than my body was out of balance. I'd been neglecting some of my own advice for a healthy life. I had to reach inwards to find a centered place where I could create my own prescription for healing. Friends were vital, but I felt challenged to come to terms with my inner fears and questions such as "Why me?" "Who will take care of me?" and a host of "What if this, or what if that, happens?" It wasn't easy. Yet doing so led me to choose activities that nourished my mind, emotions and spirit as well as my body and had a profoundly beneficial effect. I thought of myself as being on a pilgrimage—a sacred journey towards healing and wholeness.

OVER TO YOU

There was a time when cancer was generally understood to be a death sentence. That is no longer true. In the last few years, at an unprecedented speed, new avenues of research, such as the personalized medicine revolution, have led to a greater knowledge of the variety of cancers and to hopeful new treatments. However, your active participation remains key to healing. Use this practical handbook as a tool. Adapt its many suggestions to your needs and temperament, as you make decisions, follow through on treatments, organize it all in your own loose-leaf binder or notebooks and create your wellness program.

Take heart, we are now among over 14 million living Americans who are cancer survivors.

Reach Out—
Don't Go It Alone

REACH IN

1

So You've Just Been Diagnosed—What Now?

FROM THE FIRST MOMENT OF SHOCK UPON HEARING YOUR diagnosis, the earth may seem to give way under your feet and a whole range of unexpected feelings may flood through you. It is natural to fear the consequences. You may want to deny this is happening to you. You may feel paralyzed when it comes to making decisions. It is not uncommon to feel as if you are at the mercy of outside forces, or pressured by the seeming certainty of professional opinions. I certainly did. Please don't judge yourself or be ashamed of having cancer. There's no accounting for the fact that some people who do all the "right" things get cancer, while others who are not at all health conscious get off scot-free.

Don't judge yourself or be ashamed of having cancer. There's no accounting for the fact that some people who do all the "right" things get cancer.

The news may come in many ways. Perhaps you were just always tired and didn't know why. Perhaps a routine mammogram or pap smear revealed something suspicious, and after follow-up tests your doctor called you in to confirm the dreaded diagnosis. Perhaps your mother's family is known to carry a cancer gene and you have watched other relatives succumb, hoping against hope that your turn would never come. Or perhaps you suddenly found a suspicious lump.

Whether your diagnosis is conveyed to you abruptly or as kindly as possible, the impact of cancer can still, without a doubt, be like a blow to the solar plexus.

I thought I was home free—with a cancer-free or pre-cancerous condition at most when I heard my diagnosis—ductal carcinoma in situ, stage 0. My mind had quickly latched on to the last phrase of my doctor's words, "stage zero," skipping over the other medical words I didn't recognize. All my life I have understood "zero" to mean "0" or "nothing." So I relaxed and settled down with a smile on my face, expecting to hear good news about my recent biopsy. Instead, my diagnosis, DCIS for short, indicated the presence of cancerous calcifications contained within the ducts of my left breast. I was told I was "one of the lucky ones," but stage 0, I discovered, was not a cause for celebration with a "Thank God, there's no cancer." Rather, the news was conveyed with the foreboding tone of an uncertain future, implying "there appears to be no lymph involvement—yet." I became confused and wary. Apparently in medicine, "0" means something, not nothing. I was beginning to learn the language of cancer. And a wave of anger surfaced.

Apparently in medicine, "0" means something, not nothing. I was beginning to learn the language of cancer.

I had never felt the presence of a lump or problem—nor had any doctor or nurse for that matter. For years I had almost totally avoided mammograms, since some research indicates a lack of accuracy and possible radiation damage to tissue. Two years ago I had a mammogram and ultrasound with a "probably benign" diagnosis. The doctor requested that I have a follow-up mammo in six months. When I did, a year and a half later, the findings suggested a change in image. The results were still vague, but on the darker side: "Suspicious—shows an abnormality. Recommendation: further tests to be sure it is benign." For peace of mind I agreed to a biopsy. I also wanted a more conclusive diagnosis. That's how I came to be sitting in the doctor's office and how cancer—albeit in its early stage—was revealed.

Some of you may be thinking, "Well, that's no big deal." But that was when my inner turmoil and deeper journey began. Cancer is cancer, *no matter what stage it is*. Subterranean fears, I discovered, lurk all around.

Here is how my friend Donald described his experience when he first found out that cancer was suspected and later when his diagnosis was confirmed:

Donald

I came home at about five o'clock. That wasn't unusual. And I went to take a pee. That wasn't unusual either. I felt a strange kind of tugging at my bladder and the urine was bright red—blood red. That was unusual.

When I called my medical group, the doctor on call asked whether I had been injured. [No.] Had I fallen or bumped against anything? [No.] He told me to call back again in a day or two, but the bleeding completely stopped overnight. He suggested I get an I.V.P.—a process whereby they inject a radioactive dye into the blood and watch for any aberrations in the bladder. I ignored the doctor's advice. After all, the bleeding had stopped. I simply—and gladly—forgot about the whole incident. Two months later, on a visit to my own doctor for another complaint, she asked me whether I had taken the I.V.P. Hearing my negative response she declared, "You must have it. It's a test for cancer."

Cancer—the dreaded word, the disease that will not be thought of or mentioned. My mother, a physician, had died of leukemia when I was an infant. My father, a physician, had succumbed to skin cancer when I was nine. Cancer was a part of my waking nightmare.

Now it was my turn. I felt alone. I felt helpless. My mind was in a frenzy. First, there was the urologist who wanted to book surgery for me without even reading the results of the test. I had enough presence of mind to reject him. Then I found the man who would be my urologist for the next seven years. After looking at the test results, this doctor talked about the possibility of chemotherapy and suggested that only a biopsy would show how invasive the tumors were. I had to wait a long full week for the pathology report. I didn't have health insurance. At that time in New York State, no one with a pre-existing condition could get coverage. I panicked. I thought of moving to Canada, or England, or Australia or just about any place in the world that provides health care for its citizens. I felt as if I'd been hit by a ton of bricks and once, in a fleeting moment, I even thought of driving off a cliff.

Anyone diagnosed with cancer is embarking on a life-altering, bewildering, and sometimes overwhelming journey. Although there may be patterns common to all, *your* story will be different. It is important that you muster energy to become involved in your healing process, for ultimately the decisions about treatment are yours alone to make. Your health is now your top priority. Before you lies the challenge of understanding the medical and technical language of your condition and making decisions for your future health. Therein lies much growth and empowerment. Decide that you are in charge of your life, because you will undoubtedly find others—a doctor, a spouse, a friend—wanting to make decisions on your behalf, "all for the best," of course, as they see it.

It is important that you muster energy to become involved in your healing process....

In the early days following your diagnosis

- Welcome the hugs of family and friends. Let yourself be loved!
- **There is no right way to handle the news.** It is not inappropriate to watch TV, burst into tears, scream in your car or want to go for a long walk.
- It is a blessing to have someone close to you, a specially trusted family member, friend or counselor who is willing to listen to you, perhaps hold your hand and be comfortable with your tears, your confusion, fear or anger, if you experience such feelings.
- **Trust yourself.** Avoid spending time with those who try to make you talk if you don't want to, or try to get you to stop talking if you need to.
- Once you have dealt with your initial reactions, take your time to gather information and think about your choices, but also don't procrastinate making a decision. Set a "decide-by" date to aim for. Waiting too long may not be in your best interests.
- Ask yourself "What can I do to help myself become well?" instead of worrying about questions such as "Why me?"
- Read the inspiring stories of those who have survived your type and stage of cancer. Take hope that so many, in spite of a bleak prognosis from their doctor, have courageously generated their own hope and worked towards healing. See *Appendix 2* for examples.
- Write your thoughts and feelings down in a private journal as your journey unfolds.
- You may never be quite the same again. This is a life-challenging journey. Through it you may discover unexpected strengths within you. **Be gentle and kind to yourself.**

"Never try to go it alone" are the words perhaps most frequently passed on from those who have already made this journey.

When you are ready, continue to Chapter 2, which helps you to begin to put your personal support team in place. "Never try to go it alone" are the words perhaps most frequently passed on from those who have already made this journey. With others to back you up, you will be in a better position to put your medical team in place and deal with all that follows.

2

Rx. Love!
Personal Support
From Your Family,
Friends and Community

WELCOME THE SUPPORT OF TRUSTED FAMILY MEMBERS AND FRIENDS

As YOU PROGRESS THROUGH SOME OF THE UNEXPECTED twists and turns of cancer and its treatments, I hope you will allow yourself to receive the comfort and strength that others can give you. Cancer is not a shameful thing. Its causes may be multiple, especially in these days of environmental toxicity. Even if you are a very private person and you don't want your diagnosis to be widely known, consider asking for support from a very few trusted family members and/or friends who love you. Make your *own* choice about when and with whom you will share your diagnosis. You may want to ask those with whom you have entrusted your news not to spread the word until, or unless, you are ready. That's your call.

Puja   *I can't imagine what this journey would have been like without my support circles. Some friends talked with me, helped me clarify what I needed to know prior to a consultation, accompanied me to medical visits, encouraged me to get a second opinion, and pointed me in the direction of research and options. Others listened to me, invited me for a meal, or gave me a healing massage or energy balancing. They recognized my wish to make choices in keeping with my understanding of holistic health. They brought comfort as I struggled to decide what I felt would be best for my body.*

I can't imagine what this journey would have been like without my support circles.

One moment I wished I'd never had that mammogram, ultra-sound, and biopsy. Another, I wished I could just cave in and hand my health entirely over to a doctor's suggestions. It would have been so much easier. Although my head was spinning, I knew I couldn't do that. Cancer had become a wake-up call to more than I ever imagined.

How Your Family and Friends Can Help You

People generally want to DO something when someone they love is in crisis. Let them! Sometimes they may need direction from you. Do not be shy in asking for help, delegating tasks or re-directing efforts that don't appeal, or seem inappropriate, to you.

Stop saying, "I don't need help." Instead, have a wish list of suggestions beside your phone so that when someone asks you how he or she can help, you won't draw a blank.

If you have been an independent person and now find yourself facing limitations, this may be difficult for you. Stop saying, "I don't need help." Instead, have a wish list of suggestions beside your phone so that when someone asks you how he or she can help, you won't draw a blank. You can scan your list and offer an appropriate suggestion—go for errands, help with laundry, mow the lawn, look something up on the Internet, or send out an email to update friends on your progress.

If you are usually a "giver," practice receiving graciously. There will be times when you will welcome practical support—someone to arrange childcare or cook a meal. At other times you may need emotional support—someone who can listen to you and perhaps talk with you, make suggestions or hold you if you need to cry. Having a team of people with whom you can talk enables you to spread your need so that no one is overly burdened. Thus you can choose to speak to a different friend on Monday, Tuesday, Wednesday and so on.

In situations where you don't feel you can go the whole way with any course of treatment, or where you sense you are not being heard by professionals or friends, you may have to fight for what you want. Members of your team can validate your right to be heard. They can also help you clarify what you want to say or help sort out a doctor's, a spouse's or a friend's wishes from your own.

Always ask someone to accompany you to medical appointments.

Put a Personal Support Team Together

Make sure you choose people who support your philosophy of healing and medical treatment. If you suspect someone who wants to help you might give you a hard time in any way, (e.g. because they think they know what's best for you), acknowledge their help but don't invite them to be in your inner circle.

Should you wish to consider alternative treatment options, it is doubly important that your support team includes members who will appreciate your perspective and back you up. It is not good for you to have your team composed of people who fear that you'll be jeopardizing your health and your life if you do not choose a traditional medical route. The fears of your friends, family or doctor regarding your choices may be expressed to you in subtle undercurrents or blatant remarks. You want to trust your team to be open to share their informed and truthful responses but not undermine or control you.

- Once you have selected your team players, weave an approach that suits your needs and perspectives and uses their unique skills.

- Ask members of your team to offer suggestions for how they would like to be involved. You may be in for some pleasant surprises and unexpected gifts. However, don't be upset when someone is not able to respond immediately to a request you have made. They may have commitments you are unaware of. Cut them some slack and don't take it personally.

- If it becomes too difficult for any reason for someone to be on your team, release that person with gratitude for what they have been able to do.

- Select a spokesperson to keep in touch with your team for those times when you don't feel like talking or when you need some privacy.

Several months after her diagnosis my friend Esther wrote:

Esther   *I am closer with my husband and son now. We all seem to have simultaneously realized that we don't want to squander precious time holding back our appreciation for each other. My friendships too have changed. Most have deepened, yet some have parted. New ones are now in resonance with the well-being I am focusing on. I've become very close with a few other women who are also healing from breast cancer. We are a very strong support group for each other and empower each other.*

FIND GROUP AND COMMUNITY SUPPORT

Be your own best friend: get involved and informed. Several studies show, without a doubt, that patients who participate in groups do much better than those who don't.

To connect with people who have been through or are going through a similar experience, inquire about local cancer support groups. A national cancer organization may have a local chapter or contact in your area. A local hospital or treatment center may have an oncology support program. Some have trained volunteers who are willing to accompany you to appointments as "navigators." Others offer informal groups for cancer patients. I was very fortunate to be put in touch with two incredible resources in my area: an oncology support program at a local hospital and an organization that provided information about treatment options.[1] The women who founded these groups knew from personal experience what I was facing, had conducted in-depth research on breast cancer and now help patients. Both women recognized my struggles and immediately responded to me, coming with me to key medical visits. I valued their support along with the caring of close friends.

Diana was diagnosed with stage 2 breast cancer in December 1986, with twenty-two positive nodes.

I didn't feel isolated and alone with my struggles; this group gave me information, hope, and confidence....

Diana *I was very discouraged. My doctors told me they stopped counting at that number because they were so jumbled together. I followed mainstream protocols including a mastectomy and six months of chemotherapy treatments. Extremely helpful to me was a women-with-cancer support group at a women's health center in my hometown. About eight of us met every Wednesday morning to laugh, cry, inform, and express our fears and hopes with each other. The facilitators both had breast cancer themselves and they were wonderfully skillful in helping the group to bond and help each other in the most meaningful ways. I still remember this group with the greatest fondness and tears of gratitude because it made so much difference to me. I didn't feel isolated and alone with my struggles; this group gave me information, hope and confidence that I could meet the challenge of each day as it came. They were supportive fellow travelers along a rocky road. I also found I could share my experience to help others. Would I have made it without these wonderful women? I'm not sure.*

- Ask your friends if they can connect you with someone who has experienced a similar diagnosis. Cancer survivors can be a great source of emotional support and personal information, especially if they are willing to share hints that helped them cope with the downside of cancer and treatment-related symptoms such as fatigue, nausea, and other side effects described in Chapter 4. About a year into her treatment when her hair was pretty skimpy, Diana met a woman at a workshop who had had thirty positive nodes. This woman was alive and well after many years, so Diana's hope soared. Now eighteen years later, Diana herself is encouraging others. "Every one of those years has felt like a bonus and a gift," she says.

- A support group doesn't have to be comprised of people who get together in person; you can connect in other ways—now primarily through the Internet. Consider joining an online group. For example, the Association of Cancer Online Resources (www.ACOR.org) is an excellent source of support groups for all kinds of cancer. You can join a chat group where people with the same interests exchange views or a 'list serve'—an email sent to people who ask to be on its distribution list. If you ask for the information to be sent to you in a daily digest form, it will save you from reading through lots of individual emails.

- Start your own group. When Jan found her local group too negative, she went to a retreat for cancer patients in California and while there formed a support group with seven participants from around the U.S. They stayed in touch via phone calls and notes and pledged to think of, and send their healing energy to, one another at 5:00 p.m. central standard time every Sunday.

- If you need more companionship, spiritual support or simply a group experience, look for a women's, men's or mixed support group, a religious or spiritual community, a meditation group or a healing circle.

When Jan found her local group too negative, she went to a retreat for cancer patients in California and while there formed a support group with seven participants from around the US.

Look for Support in Knowledge

- Start to collect resources—articles, books, and Internet resources, etc.—*at your own pace*. Some hospitals have medical libraries that are open to the public. If you have a friend who is good at researching, enlist that person's help to get information. Finding out about the various forms of cancer and the best treatments available can be very time consuming for a novice.

- Check Chapter 6 and *Appendix 2* for more resources and ideas.

I quickly learned to become selective in my conversations with others and double check sources of information.

Puja   I visited libraries, read, contacted cancer survivor friends and colleagues, and searched the Internet for relevant research and complementary resources. It was very hard work, extremely time-consuming and quite overwhelming. I came up against another recurring problem. Everyone and every resource presented opinions—different opinions! Some research contradicted other findings. Some research was even questionable. What and whom could I trust? I quickly learned to become selective in my conversations with others and double check sources of information. It again became abundantly clear: I could not face all this alone.

Create a Personal Notebook

- Choose a blank journal, notebook or three-ring binder with loose-leaf paper to become your personal notebook.

- Use the questions in the following exploration worksheets to help you focus on the support you wish to have.

- Record your sense of what you need from others, how others have offered to support you, ideas and useful leads from informal conversations, dating each entry as you go along.

Use these questions when you are deciding how you'd like your family, friends and community to support you.

1. What are my needs?

- What *practical* support do I most need at this time?
- What *emotional* support do I most need at this time?
- What *spiritual* support do I most need at this time?
- What would NOT be of help to me?
- What might I learn to accept gracefully from others, if offered?
- What takes courage on my part to request from others?

2. How can my family and friends help me meet these needs?

- What are the strengths of my close family members and friends?
- Who is good at doing what?
- On hearing my diagnosis, what have my family members and friends offered to do, if anything?
- How would I like them to be involved?
- Would I benefit from having someone in a special role such as passing on information to other team members?

3. What other community support is available and/or would I like?

- For instance: a support group, a patient group, Internet chat group…

4. Review your responses to *all* the questions above, and then make decisions.

- List those whom you want to be on your team.
- Prioritize your needs and list who can best do what.

Take action

Now you are ready to follow through on your choices.

- Invite those you have chosen.
- Ask for what you need.
- Delegate.

Along the Way

- **Note any significant suggestions from personal conversations or emails:**

    Contact with_____(name of person)

    On _____ (date)

    About_____(topic discussed)

    Include:

    - New ideas/information
    - I'll follow-up by_____

If you receive a helpful email, print it out and insert it in your binder.

3

Harness the Power of Professional Support— Your Doctors and Healthcare Practitioners

CHOOSING PROFESSIONAL HELP

C ANCER DOESN'T HAPPEN OUT OF THE BLUE, although a diagnosis often does. It's an on-going process. Throughout life, when cells wear out, new healthy cells are constantly replacing them. For various reasons this does not always happen as it should. Occasionally abnormal cells grow that cause cancer. By the time cancer is spotted, these mutated cells have replicated out of control, because the immune system (your body's defense system) has failed to clean them up efficiently. You may have one or more of over a hundred different types of cells that can include a frequently diagnosed cancer (breast, lung, ovarian and prostate) or a more rare form. Whatever the type, you need professional help for an accurate diagnosis, advice on treatment and for treatment itself.

Most professionals want to do their best to help you heal, and many are willing to form a healing partnership with you. Choosing members of your professional team may be more complex than choosing your personal team, which is made up of friends and family whom you know and trust. In putting your professional team together, you are probably meeting doctors for the first time, on their turf, under the stress of illness. In their offices, they may appear to have a lot of power and you may feel you have very little. This perception can add to your stress and fear. You may not know much about them, and they may ask you to make quick decisions based on their diagnoses and treatment suggestions.

You can, however, be clear about the kind of partnership you wish to have. Many doctors assume that it is in your best interest to abide by the suggestions they make, without considering other possibilities. That's fine if that's what you want. If it's not, be ready to speak up, with the help of the person accompanying you to appointments. Choose a doctor who is knowledgeable, listens to you and discusses your goals. Ideally you should come away with some sense of hope, not just with tension, despair or fear.

Choose a doctor who is knowledgeable, listens to you and discusses your goals. Ideally you should come away with some sense of hope, not just with tension, despair or fear.

Your primary physician and oncologist, if solely trained in the Western "allopathic" tradition, will routinely steer you towards mainstream treatments—usually surgery and/or chemotherapy, radiation and other drugs. They may not acknowledge any other course of treatment or the integration of complementary modalities. Your health insurance company may do the same. On the other hand you will almost certainly learn from friends, neighbors and other sources, including the media, about many different treatments for cancer. Some may come highly recommended. Others may seem quite bizarre. Keep an open mind so that you do not narrow your treatment possibilities too soon. However, you may reach a point when you have to protect yourself from being overwhelmed by an avalanche of well-meaning personal anecdotes about this or that cure. Do your homework, sleep on it and then go back to it. That will help you tap into your intuition and inner knowing as well as engaging more critical thinking when you sort through all the information.

KNOW YOUR OPTIONS BEFORE YOU DECIDE

Before you sign up with a doctor or embark on a course of treatment it is wise to make your own inquiries about the providers and treatment options available. The help you need may or may not be in your own back yard, so if you are able to travel, consider how far you are willing to go. For example, when I was looking for a second opinion I cast my net wider by making inquiries about physicians in the nearest metropolitan area. Others travel further for a highly recommended specialist. You can consult an organization whose purpose is to research recommendations for cancer patients regarding the best possible resources, clinicians, treatments and locations for specific types of cancer.[1] As early as possible find out as much as you can absorb about what to expect from different approaches, professionals and institutions.

CURRENT CANCER CARE

UNDERSTANDING AND TREATING CANCER FROM DIFFERENT PERSPECTIVES

At the risk of oversimplifying, until recently there have been two main types of providers following two distinct sets of cultural and philosophical beliefs, generally practicing separately from each other. The first is mainstream or conventional Western medicine. The second is holistic healthcare within which can be found many complementary medical and alternative care modalities. Now a third possibility is emerging, known as "integrative medicine," in which an active partnership is being forged between the first and second for the benefit of the patient.

Detailed descriptions of practitioners, diagnostic tools and possible treatments of both conventional medicine and complementary care follow the bird's eye overview. For balance, take each into account. If you are well versed in Western medicine but not complementary and alternative modalities, or vice-versa, please quickly review the specific information you already have and focus on the information that is new to you. As you do this, you will begin to get a sense of your preferences—conventional, complementary and alternative, both, or integrative, if it's available.

A bird's
eye view of
current
cancer care

1. Conventional Mainstream Approach: Western Physicians

1. Focuses on specific parts of the body, with specialists trained in specific fields.
2. Primarily addresses the physical symptoms or complaints of a patient.
3. Does well with extreme, acute conditions.
4. Uses modern technology, which includes surgery, radiation and hi-tech procedures such as bone marrow and stem cell transplants. (See Chapter 11, Section 2)
5. Makes use of synthetic substances—chemotherapy, drugs and hormone blockers/therapies.

This is also known as **allopathic medicine** or **allopathy**.

2. Holistic Healthcare Approach And Its Practitioners

1. Looks at the whole person and the dynamic relationship of body, mind, emotions and spirit.
2. Looks for underlying causes or meaning of symptoms.
3. Does well with many chronic conditions.
4. Reclaims ancient ways and simpler forms of a nature-based approach.
5. Uses natural and organic substances such as herbs, vitamins, minerals and whole foods.

These providers are often referred to as practicing **complementary medicine** and/or **alternative care**.

3. Emerging Approach: Combining Mainstream Medicine And Holistic Care

1. Aims to combine the best and most appropriate of both perspectives in creative partnerships.
2. Draws on expanding research in both fields.

Physicians who have been trained in the practice of both mainstream and complementary medicine generally use the term **integrative medicine**.

The details of each follow:

1. Conventional Western Medicine

Physicians are likely to move as fast, and frequently as aggressively, as possible to eradicate cancer cells through surgery, chemotherapy and radiation. Research is focused on techniques becoming more precise, less toxic and more personalized.

Who are the mainstream cancer doctors or oncologists?

Medical oncologists treat cancer with chemotherapy, hormone therapy or biological agents.

Pathologists diagnose abnormal changes in tissues and organs by using a microscope.

Radiation oncologists treat with radiation (X-rays).

Radiologists interpret x-rays and related imagery such as ultrasound, MRI and CT.

Surgical oncologists use surgery and robotic surgery.

What are the primary mainstream treatments for cancer?

Adjuvant therapy refers to radiation, chemotherapy or hormonal therapy used in addition to the primary form of treatment, generally surgery. **Neo-adjuvant** therapy is radiation and chemotherapy treatment prior to surgery to shrink the tumor.

Chemotherapy uses drugs to kill malignant cells, preventing further growth. **Hormonal therapy** blocks hormones with drugs such as Tamoxifen or aromatase inhibitors; can also remove or add hormones.

Immunotherapy enlists patients' own immune system to fight a tumor, e.g. monoclonal antibodies.

Irradiation treats with x-ray, radioisotope, ultraviolet or infrared rays.

Radiation/radiotherapy can be used prior to surgery to shrink a tumor, given as one dose during surgery, and more often after surgery to eliminate and prevent the growth of any stray cancer cells. (Some low-dose radiation can diagnose disease; high doses can treat disease.)

Surgery cuts out the cancerous tissue.

How do mainstream practitioners come to their treatment decisions?

A biopsy removes tissue for microscopic examination and diagnosis in different ways. For example, a core needle biopsy uses a small cutting needle to remove a core of tissue; a needle biopsy uses a thin wire under x-ray control to extract cells or bits of tissue. (Local anesthesia is usually used).

An excisional biopsy is the surgical removal (excision) of an abnormal area of tissue, (an entire lump) usually along with a margin of healthy tissue, while **an incisional biopsy** removes a portion of an abnormal area of tissue, by cutting into (incising) it.

Blood sample analysis can provide crucial information by identifying, for example, white and red blood cell count and tumor markers to track the progress in treatment.

Bone marrow test/aspiration shows if there are cancer cells in the bone marrow.

Genetic analysis of a tumor can lead to more targeted therapy.

Palpating an area of concern: Manual exam with varying amounts of pressure is a preliminary way (by a patient or doctor) to determine if there are any changes—such as a lump, abnormal tissue mass, strange sensation or pain.

Radiographic Studies: X-Ray is a high-energy form of radiation. X-rays form an image of body structures by traveling through the body and striking a sheet of film. **Breast X-rays are called mammograms.**

Scans: E.g. bone scan; **Cat Scan** and **CT Scan** provide a cross-sectional view of the entire body through X-ray, which might show cancer or metastases earlier and more accurately than other imaging methods; **PET** scan (Positron Emission Tomography) can search for cancer anywhere in your body and tell you whether a tumor is benign or malignant; **MRI** (Magnetic Resonance Imaging) uses magnetic waves to create detailed pictures inside the body, providing anatomical and functional information.

Scopes: Modalities that view specific areas inside the body such as bronchoscopy (lungs) and colonoscopy (colon).

Ultrasound uses sound waves to produce images of body tissues.

As Many People, As Many Choices: About Our Stories—and Yours

The stories of our choices throughout this chapter vary greatly. Some of us opted to use only mainstream protocols. Many blended both conventional and complementary therapies in different ways. Others chose to start with mainstream, then transferred to complementary or alternative modalities, while others began with complementary and later sought out more aggressive mainstream protocols.

An appropriate choice for one person may not be valid for another. Our vignettes are intended to illustrate the varied challenges and issues facing cancer patients. **Please do not take our choices to imply in any way that you should follow in our footsteps, or use a story as evidence for a specific treatment plan.**

Each person is unique. Discuss with your physician and health care team the need for tests or the implications of test results and possible treatment plans for your own situation.

Lilly
Entirely
mainstream

) Our stories:
mainstream

Lilly made a conscious choice to trust her mainstream doctors entirely. She had confidence in the treatments they recommended. She didn't want to live with the uncertainty of wondering if she should be doing something different. In fact, she wanted to go back, as much as could be possible, to the time before she was sick when her life was "normal" and she visited a doctor once a year, not once a week. She created a box around her illness so she could ignore it except when the doctors intruded into her world. This technique kept her from dwelling on the disease and helped her to focus on the good parts of her life. To do that she had to tell herself, "I'm not sick—this is a temporary condition," and "I don't want to know much about what is wrong with me because the details are too scary for me to think about." She understood that her choice was related in some way to using denial as a means of dealing with her illness but she felt it was very effective for her and also for her other friends who have found themselves in a similar situation. She did become surprised at the seemingly endless number of doctors that are required to treat this disease. "Enough already!!" she said.

She created a box around her illness so she could ignore it except when the doctors intruded into her world.

Marty
Mostly mainstream

When I was young, cancer was one of those words I did not even like to hear. If I came across an inevitable article delineating symptoms, I would search my body and its reactions for the merest hint of their presence. One day, decades later, when I had retired I found a hard lump in my groin. My home doctor calmly asserted that we should wait two weeks and see what developed. On the return visit he looked again, noted that the lump did not move and advised me there was a 50-50 chance that it was serious. I went through both needle and surgical biopsies. The results were positive.

I had always envisioned myself collapsing into a spasm of uncontrollable fear were I to receive such news. That did not happen. I didn't dance for joy or fall back on disingenuous philosophies of reassurance but neither did I dissolve into quivering apprehension.

A gaggle of medical visits, blood draws, X-rays, CT-scans and MRI's ensued. I guess laughter helped as, for the most part, my wife and I laughed quite a bit at the comic wigs and gaudy kerchiefs I tried on, in expectation of effects from the chemotherapy I was to undergo.

I don't think that this experience broadened me or made me more sensitive. It happened and I luckily found doctors who battled my cancer and have kept it in remission for some years now. I was fortunate that the lymphoma proved treatable. I am grateful for those good years but I battled nothing. Those who treated me and those who researched and discovered treatments battled for me.

I guess laughter helped as, for the most part, my wife and I laughed quite a bit at the comic wigs and gaudy kerchiefs I tried on, in expectation of effects from the chemotherapy I was to undergo.

Puja
Mainstream initially

On hearing my cancer diagnosis, I wanted to learn about all my options. After all, I'd benefited from all kinds of healing interventions, both Western and Eastern. I assumed I would be encouraged by the doctors to review all possible treatment plans before making any decision. To my surprise and disappointment, that was not the case.

From the moment I was tagged with cancer, I began to sense that I was entering a world of subtly projected fear and not so subtle pressure. Even stage "0" had become a passport to treatment by surgery, followed by the hormonal agent Tamoxifen and radiation. In my case chemotherapy was not recommended, but there was never a hint of any other treatment plan. Making my decisions was very difficult in the face of such a set protocol by "experts." I had to gather my courage to look at all my options and then decide.

To cut or not to cut was my first dilemma. Feeling pressured to make a quick decision, I found my mind caught in the middle of a clash between the two different systems I have described—the official medical approach which would treat with aggressive localized action (surgery) and the holistic model which would attempt to treat the cancer systemically as a whole in a variety of less intrusive ways (e.g. hands-on healing, nutrition, prayer, and visualizations). I felt very uncomfortable about being asked to choose the former without any recognition of the contribution of the latter. It was as if I were a tiny speck on the horizon, increasingly being sucked into the pathway of a big machine. I feared it would run me over.

After much research and soul searching, I decided to have surgery. I was indeed very fortunate that the entire day of my surgery was very nurturing. It was a good experience from all perspectives. One friend drove me to our local hospital in the next town. I assured her it was OK to leave me. I was feeling calm, knowing that my friends, who were aware of the date and time of my surgery, were praying for me. The nurses were warm and friendly as they guided me through the preparation steps. Before I knew it, I was sitting up on a bed ready to go. Brief morning prayers came over the intercom followed by a visit from a pastoral counselor who asked if I would like her to pray with me before I was wheeled off. Although she was a Catholic (probably a nun), she knew from my registration form that I was not. Her prayer was a most beautiful inclusive sharing. She prayed for my healing in whatever way was right for me. Again, I felt surrounded by love.

It was a pleasant surprise that the nurse, who had taken my vital statistics on the pre-op day, greeted me like an old friend when she joined our little entourage in the hallway en route to the operating room. The anesthesiologist introduced himself and assured me that he knew my request was to have as little anesthesia as possible. The O.R. was much bigger and much, much colder than I imagined it. I remember asking for, and being given, blankets to keep my lower body warm. Of course it made sense when the doctor told me that a low temperature minimizes bacterial infection. As the surgeon and her team connected with me, they explained some of the preparations. Their coordination and teamwork were very reassuring. I found it paradoxical that in the most, necessarily, sterile of places I was clearly being treated with such consideration. Then I was "out."

When I came out of the recovery room, my friend welcomed me. She had been impressed and relieved that the surgeon had already taken time to tell her of the success of the surgery. She drove me to friends in my hometown. I was tired but not at all nauseous. I was very blessed that this part of my journey was so easy. By the time we reached their home, I was ready to bask in their love, and

It was a pleasant surprise that the nurse, who had taken my vital statistics on the pre-op day, greeted me like an old friend when she joined our little entourage in the hallway en route to the operating room.

eat their delicious food. I was glad that the surgery was over and relieved that the pathology slides indicated that the surgeon had gotten it all. I was very thankful for the skill and the humanity of the medical team I experienced that day.

Linda
Different mainstream treatments

Linda has been a spiritual seeker and disciple for more than twenty-eight years and has always followed unique and alternative medical and healing paths. Facing cancer, she opted for the most aggressive of the traditional medical models. In January of 1999 she noticed some vaginal spotting. After testing, a suspicious lump was found on each breast and a cyst on an ovary. Her older, very blunt doctor recommended a total hysterectomy.

With her partner's support, Linda chose first to go to a surgeon for breast biopsies. The results came back with clear margins so in fact a lumpectomy had been accomplished. Radiation was recommended. After doing some research, she decided the benefits outweighed the risks and she started the treatments. Though often very tired, Linda continued to work throughout the treatments and lived with the raw burned patches that developed beneath her breast.

Knowing the dangers of ovarian cancer, she then went to see a specialist, a popular gynecological oncologist in a city, an hour and a half away. This young bright surgeon was witty and personable and he told her everything she wanted to hear—that a hysterectomy was not necessary; that the five-centimeter cyst had not changed in size from the original test in January till April (cancer would have changed dramatically); and that if a hysterectomy was ever necessary a simple trans-vaginal procedure would suffice. "Don't worry," he said, "Have a nice trip to Alaska this summer to recuperate from the radiation and we'll see you in the Fall."

Fall showed a ten-centimeter tumor. The trans-vaginal hysterectomy was scheduled immediately. This "simple" procedure took nine hours and was actually two surgeries, during which there were complications. Linda began the prescribed course of chemotherapy right away. Although extremely upset at the doctor, she got on with her life, grateful to be able to do so. Early in 2000 she was ready to put the whole experience behind her.

To make sure every base was covered, a friend recommended seeing a top gynecological oncologist in a metropolitan area who was prominent in the national ovarian cancer society, a breast cancer survivor herself, and writer on cancer. She informed Linda that the chemotherapy she had been given was not state of the art and advised a new course of chemo immediately. She said a five-centimeter cyst in any post-menopausal woman is always suspicious and must be removed and that trans-vaginal hysterectomies are never done on women who haven't given birth vaginally and or when a growth is at all suspicious. She also strongly recommended Tamoxifen. Linda changed to those new protocols.

Six years later, in 2005, Linda took the last of her Tamoxifen pills. She was healthy in every way, yet she felt she had to be more alert now that she had lost an "extra protection." Linda and her partner were both relieved to have an excellent medical team in place. Now, ten years on, she continues her spiritual practices and she's become a scholar on foods that repair DNA, help specific symptoms, and support natural immunity.

Linda now cautions, "**When in doubt, check it out**. With hindsight I should have had a biopsy immediately on the 'cyst' on my ovary. I didn't see why I should have the total hysterectomy suggested by the first doctor, so when the second MD told me not to worry, his words were very seductive. He was saying just what I wanted to hear and I ignored my niggling feelings. The bottom line is no one knows until it gets biopsied."

With hindsight, I should have had a biopsy.... The bottom line is no one knows until it gets biopsied.

Donald
His mainstream journey (cont.)

I will never again be the helpless innocent that I was when I first encountered my disease. I have learned the importance of finding caring skilled physicians, of asking for advice and support from people who have experienced similar conditions, and of discovering how to create my own treatment.

During the seven years after my first surgery for bladder cancer, I must have had eight surgeries and at least twelve cystoscopies—excruciatingly painful cystoscopies. The urologist would check me out by pushing a fiber optic tube with a light up my urethra and into my bladder. I actually learned Lamaze breathing techniques so I would suffer less. I thought this was the way it was supposed to be. I really thought this—until I changed urologists. When my regular urologist ended his association with my health plan, I was forced to look elsewhere.

With the help of a family member I located a top urological oncologist, practicing in a large medical center. He was caring, gentle and concerned. Going there was an eye-opener. As big as the facility was, from the time I was admitted I found it to be a compassionate place. The cystoscopy test was painless. I became aware that I had suffered needlessly for seven years. I had been a total innocent. My only reference had been my previous urologist. The test, however, indicated a recurrence of the tumors. Talk about mixed feelings. I was angry at having needlessly suffered agony for seven years, very relieved at the pain free procedure, and anxious about the necessary surgery.

I had often assumed that the bigger an institution is the less caring it is, and the smaller an organization the more personal and caring the attention. I was wrong. The small urological practice to which I was wedded for seven years was cold and generally uncaring, although technically correct. Now in the hands of this caring physician, I had two more cystoscopies that year, both negative. After two years I needed cystoscopies only once a year. I began a new regimen that included distilling my own water and continuing to drink at least two quarts a day. For years I was absolutely clear. Then, in May 2005, at the annual cystoscopy, there was a small tumor. In June, I had my first surgery in over seven years. It was a surprise but I was now ready for it, fully confident in this doctor and the choices I had made.

2. Complementary and Alternative Medicine

HOLISTIC HEALTH CARE

My heritage in Scotland taught me to respect the folklore traditions of herbal medicine and natural healing remedies as well as the gifts of our family doctors.

Most holistic practitioners are to be found in the fields of **complementary and alternative medicine** (**CAM** for short). Holistic practitioners emphasize the importance of treating the body, and the person, as a whole. They work patiently to detoxify the body, build up the immune system and realign the energy flow through the body. Mental, emotional and spiritual health may also be addressed. Nutrition, herbs, exercise, meditation and visualization are just a few of the techniques that may be suggested.

My heritage in Scotland taught me to respect the folklore traditions of herbal medicine and natural healing remedies as well as the gifts of our family doctors. For example, if we children walked through a patch of stinging nettles we immediately looked for the docken plant growing close by so we could lay its broad leaves on our itchy legs. Combining treatments from different sources was taken for granted.

Who are the holistic or complementary and alternative practitioners? What are their treatments of choice?

These are somewhat complex questions. Complementary practitioners could be practicing any one or more of the following modalities recognized by the National Institutes of Health (NIH), National Center for Complementary and Alternative Medicine (NCCAM).[2] It is not an exhaustive list.

Acupuncture

Alexander Technique

Aromatherapy

Ayurvedic medicine

Biofeedback

Chiropractic

Diet therapy

Environmental medicine

Health kinesiology

Herbalism

Holistic nursing

Homeopathy

Hypnosis

Internal and external Qigong

Massage therapy

Meditation

Naturopathy

Nutritional therapy

Osteopathic manipulative therapy

Reflexology

Spiritual healing

Tai Chi

Traditional Chinese medicine

Yoga

Complementary implies that the non-allopathic practitioner is working along with conventional medicine, in a cooperative manner.

Alternative indicates a practitioner who is offering a service in place of conventional Western medicine. Alternative systems might be a non-Western system such as traditional Chinese medicine or a Western one, such as naturopathy or homeopathy.

If you did not recognize all these terms, it's not surprising. Global tele-communications and international travel have given us the option of choosing many treatments that have originated in cultures beyond our shores. A few foreign words such as 'yoga' have become part of our everyday vocabulary and need no English translation. But at times it seems to me that I am in the middle of a vast gathering—a medical potpourri in which exotic healing practices from all over the world are vying for my attention. Here are some examples:

Complementary and alternative (CAM) treatments from far and wide

From indigenous peoples worldwide comes knowledge of the healing properties of plants (herbal medicine) and healing ceremonies such as sweat lodges for cleansing and detoxifying the body.

From India come Ayurveda and Yoga: Ayurveda, meaning "science of life," dates back to the ancient Vedic civilization and is now popularized by Dr. Deepak Chopra. Yoga, closely connected to Ayurveda, is designed to reduce stress, bring better alignment of the spine and greater tone to muscles, organs and internal systems, and create inner peacefulness.

From the Far East come Acupuncture, Qigong or Chi Kung, Reiki, and Jin Shin Jitsu. All are based on the ancient Chinese and Japanese understanding that a subtle energy called "Ch'i", "Qi" or "Ki", circulates through the energy pathways or meridians of the body. When this energy is flowing freely, a person is healthy and balanced. To unblock stuck energy, a reiki healer lays hands on the patient according to a specific pattern, while an acupuncturist penetrates the skin with thin metallic needles at specific places. Chi Kung, Tai Chi and other systems activate the chi through patterns of movement and exercise.

From Europe come Homeopathy and the Bach Flower Essences. Homeopathy, discovered and developed by Dr. Hahnemann in Germany, uses minute doses of natural remedies created from herbal, mineral and animal substances akin to the disease to treat "like with like." With the Bach Flower Remedies or essences, Dr. Edward Bach in England contributed significantly to the field of vibrational medicine. Their healing properties help balance emotions. For example, "Rescue Remedy," the most commonly used composite essence, as its name suggests, can help you at times of shock.

In America a number of body therapies have been pioneered. For example, Chiropractic clears subluxations, Rolfing is a deep tissue work, Rubenfeld Synergy accesses the mind-body connection through bodywork and Cranial-sacral work calls for light sensitive touch. Highly developed computer programs and complex biofeedback systems have also been birthed here.

You may find it easier to understand what is involved in complementary and alternative care by looking at the types of intervention they offer:

Alternative systems such as Chinese medicine are complete in themselves. They have often evolved in other continents apart from, or prior to, the Western model.

Body-based manipulations and adjustments such as chiropractic, release the places where you most hold tension such as the spine, neck and shoulders; massage relaxes muscle and connective tissue and helps the lymph to flow; physical therapy helps remedial rehabilitation.

Emotional release techniques, counseling and especially body-oriented psychotherapies such as Bioenergetics and The Rubenfeld Synergy Method help you get in touch with your feelings and how they have been held in your body—so that you can clear out old suppressed feelings and honor current feelings. **Expressive therapies**, such as art or music, help to open pathways of insight and get your creative juices flowing in a non-verbal manner. **Movement and exercise instruction** promote circulation, strengthen your muscles and build your stamina.

Mind-body interventions (mental strategies to influence the body) such as stress reduction and hypnosis, help you relax; guided visualizations with cancer-specific imagery can support your medical treatment. **Meditation and spiritual practices** help you to give space for your inner being and to reconnect with the miracle of life.

Natural therapies such as diet, herb, vitamin, and nutritional counseling assist in de-toxifying your liver and building your immune system.

Vibrational medicine therapies offer choices in healing that use the subtle energy field theory as the basis, such as The Bach Flower Essences, and homeopathic remedies. They include **Hands-on-energy healing techniques** to free up stuck or blocked energy, replenish depleted energy and generally help energy to flow more freely. Many are trademarked by names such as Reiki, Therapeutic Touch, Touch for Health, the Feldenkrais Method and Polarity Therapy, identifying a particular style and approach.

How do complementary practitioners come to their treatment decisions?

The methods of inquiry utilized by complementary and alternative practitioners are extremely varied, so don't be surprised if, for example, a Chinese physician holds your wrist to take and evaluate three levels of eighteen pulses as well as examining the state of your tongue; or if you are asked unexpectedly detailed questions by a homeopathic doctor. She may request an extremely lengthy life history, much more complex than the tick-off intake sheets presented to new patients almost anywhere else. She may then take copious notes as you present all aspects of your life experience (medical, social and psychological) in order to arrive at an understanding of the underlying causes.

Other examples: Some practitioners use health kinesiology to test muscles to see where there is a weakness in the body and what food, supplements, minerals and vitamins are needed to strengthen or support better functioning. Other practitioners might focus on gathering information with biofeedback systems and other extremely sophisticated high-tech machines, which use the technology of quantum physics along with advances in energy medicine to assess energetic imbalances, including cancer. Yet others might suggest you undergo screening such as digital infrared thermal imaging (thermography)[3] or go to mainstream specialists for further testing that CAM practitioners are not able, or equipped, to offer.

Remember, when you present a symptom, complementary practitioners will mainly focus on finding a root cause for the imbalance within the whole system rather than treating a specific part of the body.

Our stories: complementary and alternative

Puja

CAM after Mainstream

For decades, my practitioners of choice have included massage therapists, hands-on healing energy body workers, acupuncturists, chiropractors, naturopaths and psychotherapists. I always used complementary holistic health care to focus on preventive medicine. I lead a pretty healthy balanced life style, which includes exercise, diet and meditation, but I still got cancer!

Before and after surgery, I visited my naturopath. She included health kinesiology as a diagnostic method helpful for selecting whole foods, vitamins and supplements to balance my system. When I could, I received massage and energy balancing sessions individually or as part of a healing circle. I frequently meditated and used visualization tapes and a sauna. I became clear that having cancer in my body didn't mean that holistic care had failed me.

At the follow-up appointment after surgery, the surgeon was pleased that my scar was healing well. I gave information about the complementary support I had, but there was no hint of variation on the previously stated theme, that I should consider Tamoxifen and radiation. I don't know now why it came as a shock that I should be expected to continue to treat my body as a machine to be fixed with drugs and possible radiation without reference to other treatment options. My desire to weave a path that would include holistic healing modalities had not changed. And so at this point I chose to draw a line. I was not going to take Tamoxifen or sign up for radiation. I sought out an oncologist who might understand the holistic perspective, and I continued to work with my complementary practitioners, sorting my way through the maze of ethical, medical, emotional and personal issues that this journey stirred up.

From time to time I saw a healer who used morphology, the study of form and structure of organisms, (included in medical schools in France) as part of his assessment. After laying-on-of-hands spiritual healing, he suggested specific visualizations for me to practice several times daily to address the physical and emotional issues I needed to heal. I consulted a medical intuitive. I chose to eat more organic food. Intrigued as I always am by new cutting edge work in healing and psychology, I signed up for sessions with a practitioner trained in the use of a sophisticated biofeedback machine,[4] and I chose to start using thermography as an additional screening tool.

Some of those choices, which were natural for me, might appear strange to you. There is room for much diversity as you put your own creative plan into action.

Some of those choices, which were natural for me, might appear strange to you. There is room for much diversity as you put your own creative plan into action. Please don't imitate my choices. For example, if you have a more invasive cancer or one with more negative features, you might want to sign up for radiation and hormonal therapy.

Esther

Blending complementary and alternative treatments

After surgery to remove a tumor and some lymph nodes, I was assured by my surgeon that my "margins were clear." For follow-up treatments I chose an MD who was well known for his active involvement in complementary and alternative medicine since 1974. His approach rests on the assumption that cancer is a systemic, not a local, disease even before it reaches advanced stages. His strategy is to support and enhance the body's defense functions, to mobilize internal healing forces—to assist the body in neutralizing and/or breaking down the cancer. This was in line with my philosophy. I underwent intravenous vitamin drip treatments twice a week for three months, gradually reduced over time till it was only once per month. I also took many different supplements daily to strengthen and support my immune system.

I designed my own wellness program, using an amazing variety of other modalities—visualization, acupuncture (particularly a powerful form of acupuncture called light color puncture), a biofeedback device, and many healings from gifted intuitive healers including a healer from the Philippines and another from Haiti. I believe there were many contributing factors from the past leading to my cancer. For example, when I was young, every summer I picked and ate huge numbers of apples directly from trees, which were constantly sprayed with insecticides; I lived near a nuclear reactor and used birth control pills for many years; and I recognize I had emotional issues which contributed to my cancer. I believe I'm doing what I can to eliminate their effects and I feel stronger in many ways now.

Every six months Esther goes for a blood test to monitor for the presence of cancer. After three years, there is no cancer. We can't know which, if any, of all those treatments were useful or what would have happened if she had done nothing. The jury is still out.

Donald, as you have read, continued to rely primarily on surgery every time a regular cystoscopy indicated recurring bladder cancer.

Donald

Trying out complementary options

I decided that anything my body rejected so totally was not for me. It could be for other people but not me.

I also tried everything. I tried Aryuvedic medicine. I tried meditating on the energy chakras to bring the bladder, the area of my cancer, (second chakra) into balance. I looked at the metaphor for the illness since I can see that each illness has a message. The bladder is the area of anger—of holding anger. I started with the notion of being "pissed off" letting that lead me to a greater understanding. I even bought a wheat grass sprouter and juicer and grew my own. I found it so disgusting that I would gag each time that I tried it. After six months of that ordeal I decided that anything my body rejected so totally was not for me. It could be for other people but not me. I *began drinking at least two liters of water every day. That felt right and I have been doing so for years now.*

Following her diagnosis of non-Hodgkin's Lymphoma, Ujjala was advised to have surgery and chemotherapy. As a spiritual counselor and a person involved in the healing arts for thirty-seven years, it was hard for her to think of taking chemotherapy treatments but she recognized it was necessary. She trusted her doctor of twenty-seven years and he too advised it in addition to other complementary modalities such as iscador injections.[5]

Ujjala
Doing something different second time round

During chemotherapy treatments, I never allowed myself to think of chemo negatively. It was a chemical that I was telling my body to use in a healing way. I learned that by using both the medical and complementary worlds, I was able to heal faster. First, before surgery I went on a strict Macrobiotic diet for three months. After surgery I did very well by continuing with a simple diet, in the hospital and at home, of brown rice, miso soup and steamed veggies. While on chemo, I watched what I ate but found that my body would tell me even more than my mind what I needed to eat. For example, I craved red meat—me, who hadn't eaten red meat in 30 years, now wanted it!! And I had no problem digesting it at all. That surprised me. My body went through changes concerning food. It was like being pregnant; cravings would come and go. Sometimes I longed to eat meat, sometimes just to eat vegetables. During my treatment I had no major side effects…I ran my business with no problem, went skiing, dancing and lived a full life.

I discovered that a recurrence, no matter how scary, gave me the opportunity to take another approach.

After treatment, my joints were stiff and achy, so I did research and found the original herbal blend called Ojibwa, similar to the popular Essiac tea. It got rid of the stiffness. I also spent time building up my immune system and cleansing my body: I used various modalities such as acupuncture, laying on of hands healing, medicinal teas and, since I was always involved in indigenous sweat lodges, it was natural for me to take part in these purification ceremonies. I took saunas several times a week too. All of it contributed.

Five years later, I expected to get the usual "all clear" from a routine CT scan. Instead, I was shocked to hear that I had an enlarged lymph node near the aorta. I was told the physicians wanted to do a stem-cell transplant. This freaked me out so I tuned into my intuitive sense of what was right for me. Listening to my own body's wisdom was really important. I discovered that a recurrence, no matter how scary, gave me the opportunity to take another approach. I went for a second opinion and, after doing plenty of research, decided to try only complementary treatments in line with my gut feelings at the time. I found a doctor who suggested I use biochemical herbal supplements and detox with high colonics and other special procedures that worked the lymphatic and immune systems so my body could at least stabilize and/or heal itself. It's now ten years since my original diagnosis.

Sprinkled throughout later chapters you will find vignettes of others who also turned to guided imagery, prayer and other spiritual or "non-medical" practices, to assist healing.

Don't Give Up Hope

These days the line between Western medicine and complementary or alternative care keeps shifting as a result of public demand, as more holistic treatments are researched and accepted by mainstream medicine, and as integrative medicine takes root. Don't give up hope if you think a specific treatment is not available in your area. The pace of these changes varies greatly in different parts of the country but it is happening noticeably, so make sure you get up-to-date information as to where and to whom you can go for treatment for your type of cancer before you make any decisions.

3. Integrative Medicine

Integrative physicians use various combinations of the screening, detection and treatment tools of both mainstream and complementary medicine for which there is scientific evidence of safety and effectiveness.

As more patients and doctors experience the need for an integrative approach, a new breed of physicians trained in *both* allopathic medicine and complementary care and practicing *Integrative Medicine* is emerging from accredited medical schools. Post-graduate CAM courses for practicing doctors are also available.[6]

As this trend increases so, too, will the opportunity for you to receive this type of coordinated assessment and care without traveling long distances.

Ximena
Finding a new way to address to her concerns

Twelve years after my diagnosis, I went to hear a doctor give a public lecture about the link between the toxic load from heavy metals on the body and cancer which disturbed me. I was still fearful from time to time about a recurrence and wanted to do everything I could to prevent one. I went to see this MD who worked in an integrative manner. At his suggestion I did a 6-hour urine analysis, and found that the levels of lead and mercury in my body were off the charts. (Could it be caused by all those tuna sandwiches?!) I started a 4-month chelation therapy protocol to reduce the levels of heavy metals and have taken additional supplements daily since. It makes sense to me to take such stress out of the body and I'm blessed to have the financial resources to be able to do this.

Mary
Choosing integrative medicine

When an enlarged lymph node was located under underneath my right arm five months after surgery, I found an integrative physician who practiced Ayurveda. I was happy that he really took the 'precautionary principle' seriously, preferring to use natural non-invasive procedures. He said, "Let's see what we can do without surgery." So I went on a 21-day Ayurvedic diet and detoxification program and then received cancer treatments three times a week on a Rife machine for energy wellness.

YOUR CANCER CARE CHOICES

WHAT TO CONSIDER BEFORE GOING MAINSTREAM

You have the power to choose your professional team. It's your body! You don't need to stay with the first doctor you consult unless you have strong confidence in him or her.

You have the power to choose your professional team. It's your body!

Your general practitioner (GP), or primary care physician, is usually the first person to turn to for routine tests and for help with any troubling symptom. Thus she or he is often the person to suggest further testing and consultations that may lead to the discovery of cancer. Always ask your primary care physician to recommend more than one name for any doctor or service so that you can find the right fit.

- Make inquiries about the expertise of the professionals to whom you will eventually entrust your care, even within the limits of an existing medical insurance plan. For example, "Is the doctor board certified with excellent references?" If her manner and style of working is important to you, ask "Does she have a reputation of being brusque or patient, straightforward or ambiguous? Is he available during non-office hours with good back up coverage when off-duty?"... and so on.

- Check out organizations that research the best treatments and doctors for your type of cancer in your area, across the country or abroad, such as those in *Appendix 2*.

- When you exercise your choices regarding your surgeon, your oncologist, who to go to for a second opinion consultation, or where to go for testing, consider their hospital affiliations:

  ~ Do you have a choice of hospitals?

  ~ Do you need a local community hospital or a large medical center or teaching hospital where there is a wider range of specialists?

~ If you are in a hospital overnight or longer, will you be able to eat non-hospital food, if that is a concern?

~ Will you have access to services such as massage, patient support groups, and meditation?

~ Who is allowed to visit you and when?

Once the choice of doctor and hospital are in place, other choices such as anesthesiologist or radiologist will follow automatically.

It can be exceedingly relevant to your decision to ask yourself questions such as:

• What will my needs be if I do this treatment?

• What sort of support might I require following this treatment?

• Is this treatment within an easy distance from my home?

• How will my life be different after this treatment?

If you want to know about statistics for various kinds of treatments, don't let yourself be frightened by, or pressured into a course of treatment based solely on, such "facts." Research reports an aggregate of probabilities. It tells you what may be likely, not what will be in your case. Hidden influences can slant research and, as Albert Einstein said so well, "Not everything that can be counted counts, and not everything that counts can be counted."

A very close friend relocated to another part of the country to be near his family and to be within easy walking distance of the medical facility there.

Since a doctor cannot possibly know everything, don't expect him to be your only source of information—especially about complementary treatments outside his field unless he has received CAM or integrative training. When I asked about nutrition, the answer shot back, "I'm a doctor. I don't know about that." How much more reassuring it would have been to have been told, "That isn't my area of expertise, so let me recommend this book—or that nutritionist." However, later I realized that I wouldn't expect my naturopath to be familiar with all the mainstream cancer protocols either. From time to time patients have the opportunity to inform and thus educate doctors about complementary resources while others may inform and educate complementary practitioners about state-of-the-art Western treatments.

What to Consider Before Going Complementary

Although most cancer patients choose to follow mainstream protocols, a large number also seek an extensive range of complementary care, with or without the active support of their doctors.

You have the power to choose your professional team. It's your body! You don't need to put yourself in the hands of the first complementary care practitioner you consult unless you have strong confidence in her or him.

Many suggestions listed in *What to consider before going mainstream* are also relevant when you are considering complementary treatments, such as:

• Ask for more than one referral.
• Make inquiries as to the practitioners' expertise, training, manner and management style.
• Check out organizations that research the best protocols for your type of cancer.

Complementary practitioners usually do not specialize in seeing only cancer patients as a Western oncologist does because their emphasis in on treating the whole person. Most have some cancer patients in their practice. You may want to ask the extent of their experience working with cancer patients.

The training of Western mainstream doctors is extensive, highly regulated and rigorous. So is the training of many holistic healthcare practitioners such as naturopaths, osteopaths and homeopaths. Although less extensive, some other modalities, such as chiropractors and massage therapists, undergo rigorous training. Many states have regulating bodies. If you are in doubt about a complementary professional's training credentials and length of experience as a practitioner, and licensure, it may be even more essential to check out websites and directories of professional organizations. Some complementary traditions can call on thousands of years of experience and knowledge. The contribution of these healing traditions from ancient ways of knowing is now being given more recognition by the established medical community, but more understanding, supervision and integration are needed.

In some modalities, lesser-trained people can practice without supervision. Many do good work and bring much love to their sessions. This in itself can contribute to healing, but caution is advised before you put yourself in the hands of an unknown practitioner whose reputation you do not know or cannot check out.

There's an immense amount of fear surrounding the big C—CANCER—seeping through the pores of our culture. You may feel it even more if you dare depart, sometimes even in the slightest, from the path most traveled. Don't expect encouragement from your mainstream physicians if you choose to explore the contribution of complementary medicine. Enlist ongoing support to help you deal with, and then stay clear of, your fear as much as possible. Sometimes, as Franklin D. Roosevelt said during World War II, "The only thing we have to fear, is fear itself."

Don't expect your complementary practitioners to be knowledgeable and up-to-date about mainstream protocols.

WHAT TO CONSIDER BEFORE GOING INTEGRATIVE

You have the power to choose your professional team. It's your body!

You have the power to choose your professional team. It's your body! You don't need to put yourself in the hands of the first integrative practitioner you consult unless you have strong confidence in her or him.

- Review the suggestions listed in the previous two sections.
- If integrative medicine is important to you, look for a physician who works as part of a team with holistic practitioners. Or look for physicians with dual qualifications. They could be licensed for both. For example, as an MD and an ND (naturopathic doctor) or an MD and an LAc., (licensed acupuncturist.) In integrative medicine, a second qualification is not just tacked on as an optional extra, but indicates that the physician has made a conscious choice towards offering another option that works synergistically with his or her earlier training.
- Check out the availability of an integrative medical health center or integrative cancer care center connected to a hospital near you.

Other Considerations

Second Opinions

Although the phrase "second opinion" is in common usage, it is important to remind yourself that you are entitled to it. You also have the right to more than one second opinion, as many as you need, to become clear that you are on the right course. An additional expert opinion can be helpful in a number of ways. It may allay your fears and give you peace of mind. It may caution you that there is more to be taken into consideration than you have thus far been aware, or even that you might have to look for another doctor.

- If you can, get a second opinion from a doctor who trained, practices at, or is affiliated with a different medical center. That way you are more likely to get a different perspective. Consider also getting an additional opinion from a complementary practitioner. Check with your insurance company to see what your policy covers.

- If you find a doctor with excellent references in the specialty you need but who is outside your health insurance plan (as happened in my case), it can be worth paying out-of-pocket expenses for a consultation, which may add to your understanding.

- Never forego getting a second opinion because you think you might "hurt your doctor's feelings." That should not be an issue for you or your physician.

- On the other hand, don't waste time shopping around waiting until you find a doctor who tells you exactly what you want to hear. Eventually you may find someone who will do so, but that may not necessarily be the best course of action.

Professional Cooperation

- Advise your cancer doctors of any other health conditions for which you are being treated even if the secondary condition seems unrelated to your cancer.

- If you plan to combine mainstream and holistic treatments, inform your physicians of the names of your complementary or alternative practitioners and be specific about their modality, and vice-versa.

Never forego getting a second opinion because you think you might "hurt your doctor's feelings." That should not be an issue for you or your physician. On the other hand, don't waste time shopping around.

There is an extensive range of complementary practitioners, and so it is important that your health care providers are all aware of the types of treatment you are receiving. If you wish to blend the best of all possible care, if possible, select a doctor who will support your intention. A physician, as a professional, should respect your decision to see another provider offering a different modality.

At some point you may benefit from meeting non-medical personnel: an aesthetician, cosmetician, hair/wig consultant, life coach, minister/rabbi/imam, personal trainer, prosthesis maker, psychotherapist, spiritual counselor, or yoga teacher. These people can be part of your team for reducing stress and maintaining balance in all aspects of your life. (Get references from your friends, other cancer survivors, health professionals, support groups, local health magazines, Internet sites and online chat groups.)

RESEARCH

A promising line of research is often made public before the research is complete and well ahead of its actual availability. The accuracy of a medical research study depends on many factors such as its design, the number of patients involved, the definitions of "success" used, and whether or not there is a control group. Scientists usually consider valid research to be randomized, controlled, double-blind, prospective studies. Such research is expensive and when applied to medicine often requires financial backing from the government, corporate businesses such as the pharmaceutical industry or philanthropic institutions. Most research money goes to mainstream medicine and fewer studies have been set up to examine alternative or complementary therapies. As a result, many doctors are either unwilling to recommend, or feel uneasy about recommending, complementary protocols which have not been validated through research.

On the other hand, while there may not be scientifically valid research proving the efficacy of the various complementary practices, there is certainly a great deal of consistent anecdotal "evidence" that such treatments can work. Many people have been helped by modalities that have been used for centuries, especially in other countries or cultures. There is also a conundrum—it is often impossible to predict in advance which specific treatment will benefit one person but not another. Could this be accounted for by genetic factors? Or chemistry? Or trust in the modality arising from personal, cultural or religious beliefs?

Some physicians may therefore be prepared to give a qualified cautionary recommendation along the lines of "We don't know how helpful such treatments are because of the lack of hard research, but they may be useful in individual cases..."

Are Clinical Trials For You?

It is often impossible to predict in advance which specific treatment will benefit one person but not another.

Clinical trials are research studies that evaluate the effectiveness of new treatments by comparing them to standard treatments. They take place across the country in hospitals, clinics, cancer centers, pharmaceutical labs, and physicians' offices. New treatments under study might be drugs, gene therapy, immune vaccines and other advances including non-conventional approaches. If you are eligible for a clinical trial, you may be one of the first to benefit from a new treatment, while contributing to the growing body of cancer research. There could be some as-of-yet undiscovered side effects and risks involved in the new treatment; however, in the service of objectivity, you will not know whether you are receiving the new intervention or the standard treatment, but you will be closely monitored.

- To find a clinical trial appropriate to your type and stage of cancer, first ask your cancer specialist. Your doctor cannot possibly keep up with all of them, so make a search on your own since there are so many trials out there. You can go online or call a national organization. Give them the information about your type of cancer and ask for information about latest treatments, clinical trials, and financial aid.

- Select 2 or 3 studies that look promising to you. Show the summaries of these trials to your doctor. Select your first choice and devise a plan of action, including making a list of questions to ask when you make contact with the chief investigating officer of the trial.

TREATMENT RISKS

Always be vigilant to be sure you know what will be done, and why, before you begin treatment. Not only can unexpected complications to surgery occur as in Linda's case, but also some treatments may carry greater potential risks because they have to be so precisely targeted to a specific limited area of the body. Depending solely on complementary treatments, however, is not risk-free. It could result in the postponement, or lack, of critical aggressive treatment when needed. This is of great concern to mainstream cancer specialists.[7]

It is important to weigh the risks versus the benefits of any treatment suggested, including your medications. *The Nursing 2016 Drug Handbook* (or current year available) is a good resource, since information given with prescription medication is often limited. Ask your pharmacist for a printout of any medication prescribed.

WILL IT RECUR?

There are many different kinds of cancers each with varying life expectancies, prognoses and treatment plans. Many cancer survivors live a long active life. Some survivors have journeyed through several forms of the disease over an increasing number of years. No two journeys are the same. You are unique. Doctors can't tell in advance whether there will never be another trace of cancer or whether, like Donald, you'll find yourself tracking cancer on more than one journey even after the first "all-clear"—perhaps for the rest of a very long life that includes remissions.

Ujjala, whom you met on page 33, encourages, "Don't give up—especially a second or third time around. It may be a chance for you to do something in a different way."

Making Your Cancer Care Decisions

CHOOSING TREATMENT MODALITIES

Use the next three steps to clarify your preferences using both your thinking and feeling capabilities *before* you make decisions about your treatment. If this thorough approach feels overwhelming to you, just do what you can:

- Give yourself a break between steps.

- Ask a friend to go through it with you, and perhaps make a note of your answers.

- Do whatever feels useful to you in order to be ready to select your professional team (Step 4) and leave the rest.

Step 1: Ask yourself— what are my *initial* treatments preferences?

1. What kinds of diagnostic tools and interventions have worked for me in the past?

2. For my specific cancer diagnosis, what do I see to be the benefits and strengths of:

   - Western medicine?

   - Complementary and alternative care?

   - A combination of conventional and complementary modalities?

3. How confident, comfortable and hopeful do I feel treating my cancer with:

   - Recommendations and prescriptions of mainstream physicians?

   - Recommendations and prescriptions of complementary and alternative care practitioners?

   - A combination of conventional and complementary modalities?

Use the following charts to further clarify these questions.

Quickly put a check under the 'yes,' 'no,' or 'maybe' headings in order to indicate your preferences. (*Yes, I'm interested. No, I won't use. Maybe, I'm currently undecided.*) Remember this is for a quick response:

WESTERN OPTIONS

Tests	YES	NO	MAYBE
Biopsy			
Blood sample analysis			
Cat Scan or CT Scan			
Genetic testing			
Mammography			
MRI			
Palpating			
PET scan			
Radiographic studies (X-ray)			
Ultrasound			
Other			

Treatments	YES	NO	MAYBE
Chemotherapy			
Drugs			
Immunotherapy			
Irradiation			
Radiotherapy			
Surgery			
Other			

COMPLEMENTARY OPTIONS

Tests	YES	NO	MAYBE
Biofeedback			
Detailed life history			
Eye, tongue skin exam			
Muscle testing			
Pulses			
Thermography			
Other			

Treatments	YES	NO	MAYBE
Acupuncture			
Aromatherapy			
Ayurvedic			
Bach flower essences			
Biofeedback			
Chiropractic			
Energy healing			
Essential oils			
Health kinesiology			
Holistic nursing			
Homeopathy			
Massage therapy			
Meditation			
Naturopathy			

Treatments (cont.) YES NO MAYBE

	YES	NO	MAYBE
Nutritional/ herbal counseling			
Osteopathic manipulation			
Physical therapy			
Reflexology			
Spiritual healing			
Tai Chi			
Traditional Chinese medicine			
Yoga			
Other			

1. **Review your quick answers to the first impressions chart. Note where most of your pluses are. Add the pluses up for *mainstream* and *complementary* and ask:**

   Is there a pattern to my preferences? Do my first impressions guide me towards mainstream treatment, complementary care, or to a combination of conventional and complementary modalities?

2. **Now think about all the information you have thus far gained from your experience, discussions and research, and ask:**

   Given my type of cancer, do my first impressions still hold up? What is my case for going mainstream, going complementary, or for combining treatments?

   What else do I need to know before making an informed choice?

3. **Research the things you would still like to know before deciding:**

STEP 3: Sharpening your focus— towards a more considered, informed opinion

Track down information you still need from organizations that research the answers to your treatment questions, from libraries, the Internet, local support groups, or health newsletters. If needed, ask a member of your team to help you.

4. **Tap into your intuition again:**

   What is your gut feeling about each approach? Give yourself time to slow down, e.g. by walking in nature, so that you can feel your inner response to each possibility.

5. **Ask more questions such as:**

   - What is the advice of my physician and/or my CAM health provider?
   - Have I been given any choices of treatment? If needed, how can I initiate that discussion?
   - What mainstream treatments are specifically recommended for my condition? What complementary treatments are specifically recommended for my condition? What treatments are congruent with my perspectives about healing?
   - What is the evidence in support of both mainstream and complementary recommendations?
   - What do clinical trials of patients with my type and stage of cancer show about treatments recommended by my Western doctor? What is the evidence in support of these treatments?
   - What is my considered judgment now about what my body needs from conventional medicine and/or complementary care? Does my intuitive sense support these conclusions?
   - If I prefer combining treatments, **how much can I handle**? Would I prefer treatments to be concurrent or sequential?
   - How far am I prepared to travel for the treatment of my choice?

With the clarity you have gained in steps 1-3, use Step 4 to help you select the physicians and other providers you need.

1. List your preferred modalities for treatment.

   List the professionals, such as your GP, who are already part of your team and in whom you already have confidence. Note the field of expertise of each.

   What different professional skills do you need to add to your team? e.g. an oncologist? an acupuncturist? Now? Later?

2. Review Chapter 3 and make a list of important criteria for your choice of doctor (e.g. training, distance, openness to other team members etc.):

   Make sure that doctors you choose are "Board Certified" in their specialty.

3. Do you feel hopeful, supported and compatible with each of the practitioners you wish to choose? If you don't have a positive sense, reconsider your choice.

4. If you need more information, have you—

   - Asked your general practitioner and other practitioners for recommendations?
   - Checked out national directories and referral services?
   - Asked your friends for references?
   - Asked local cancer survivors?
   - Checked out websites?

5. As you make the necessary arrangements with each professional, add their contact information to your own *Yellow Pages*. (See Appendix 1)

STEP 4: Time to choose your professional team

Record your feelings and responses in your journal or notebook throughout this time. Expressing yourself in writing is a good way to keep coming back to what is important.

Coordinating Your Treatment

A health care provider is generally needed to receive and coordinate all your health reports and tests from your other health care specialists—such as your surgeon, oncologist, radiologist, radiation oncologist, plastic surgeon, hospital social worker and complementary or integrative practitioner.

- Consider who you would like to undertake the responsibility of overseeing your total treatment plan. Your primary physician is often the most appropriate choice for conventional cancer care. Choose someone you are comfortable with. If that person is not able to do so, ask for another referral.

If you can't find such a willing person, then this book will be a resource to help you be your own overseer— and your own advocate. Take this book or your copy of *My Hope & Focus Cancer Organizer* with your notes and questions to appointments as a reminder that cancer care can be a coordinated service.

4

Get the Most Out of Your Appointments

Before Appointments

PREPARE THOROUGHLY

ONCE YOU HAVE YOUR SUPPORT SYSTEMS IN PLACE, THE next step is to focus on treatment-related visits. The more you prepare for health-related appointments, the more you will get out of them. While it is normal to feel overwhelmed, being well prepared will build your confidence. It is helpful to list in advance all the questions you wish to ask, whether your appointment is an initial consultation or a follow-up visit at any stage along the way.

Plan ahead to invite a member of your personal support team or a local advocacy group, if there is one, to go with you to help you stay focused during your appointments. It is well researched that when we are stressed, our memory is less sharp and we are more likely to "space out." We may be tempted to give away our power to someone in authority and thus acquiesce prematurely or agree to something we would not choose under normal circumstances. That's why having an advocate or companion is so important.

Before you meet a practitioner who has given you a diagnosis, or from whom you wish to get a diagnosis or a test result, ask yourself, "What do I want to know?"

- Connect more fully with what you want to ask or say by taking a few slow deep breaths.
- Make a list of your questions and concerns.

First steps

- Review, reorder and regroup your questions and concerns according to the following six key categories of questions:

  1. What exactly is my diagnosis?

  **2. What does my diagnosis mean?
  Or, what do the results of this test mean?**

  3. What are my treatment options?

  4. What are your specific recommendations?

  5. What is the timing of recommended treatments?

  6. What about_____? (List other concerns)

- Go through the list systematically to make sure that you have left nothing out and to check if the wording could be more precise.

- If you are not sure what to ask, check out Examples 1–6.

- Be as detailed and clear as possible. It's your right to have your questions answered. It's your body and your life!

- Make extra copies of the list to take with you to your appointment, one for the person accompanying you and one for your physician or health professional, if you wish him or her to have it.

- **Respect the limits of what you can comfortably handle at any one time as you do this preparation. Take breaks and enlist help so that you don't get overwhelmed.**

I discovered it was very important to be as detailed and clear as possible.

Physicians are very busy people who are often pushed to their limits. Understandably, they may not want to take the time to get the gist of what you want to say if you waffle around, keep repeating yourself or are reluctant to give them information. Some physicians welcome a fax or email of your questions and concerns prior to a visit, especially if you are referring to something you want them to read. If you know the doctor would like to see such a list, fax it to his office. In either case, the squeaky wheel most often gets the grease, so be ready to speak up.

Select Your Own Detailed Questions

The first series of questions, *Examples 1–6*, shows you how to expand upon each of the six main categories pertaining to diagnosis, possible treatment options, your doctor's recommendations and general issues.

The second series, *Examples 7–10*, will be useful when you are preparing to meet a practitioner about *specific* treatment interventions or follow-up tests. Adapt these questions for *your* type of cancer and for other treatments, such as radiation.

Select only those questions that are important to you for a specific visit. In each case, cross-out questions you do not wish to ask and add your own.

....

1. What exactly is my diagnosis?

Regarding diagnosis and possible treatment

- Can you tell me the possible causes for these specific symptoms_____? What tests were used? What specific information did the test show?

- Could there be other reasons for my symptoms?

- How did you arrive at your opinion? How certain are you?

- Please describe my condition in simple language.

- What is the size of the malignant area in centimeters?

- What is the grade of cells (aggressiveness of cells)? Do you already know this from the lab test; if not, when will you know?

- Are they fast moving, or slow moving? Hard to destroy, or easy to destroy? Hard to remove, or easy to remove? And are there supportive tests that can tell me more about my tumor, e.g. estrogen receptor status?

- Has the cancer spread to any other site? If so, where?

- What other sites have been checked for cancer and found cancer free?

2. What does my diagnosis mean?

- How will this diagnosis affect my life? Do I have to make any changes day to day?

- What must I now take into consideration?
- Do I need further tests? Is the test you are recommending necessary to identify the type of cancer I have? Will this test help you (the doctor), or me, come to a more informed decision? What will these tests entail?
- What are your specific recommendations regarding next steps?
- If a mainstream doctor is recommending a test, do I want or need any diagnostic tests from a different viewpoint? If so, what complementary or alternative diagnostic tools are in line with my perspectives about healing?
- If a complementary practitioner is recommending a test, which one, and why? Have I checked that it is not a duplication of a test already suggested by my mainstream doctor?

3. What are my treatment options?

- Is this _____ a standard treatment? Have you had success with this treatment?
- Are there alternatives? If so, what?
- How does a practitioner decide which treatments to recommend? What is the evidence for your recommendations?
- For each possible option, please tell me where the treatment will be given. What is the duration of the treatment? How often will it be given?
- What side effects are likely, and/or possible? How do I deal with them and with any pain?
- What are the possible risks? Short-term? Long-term?
- Do you know of any experimental treatments? Are there any clinical trials for my kind of cancer? Would I be eligible to participate? What are your recommendations regarding experimental treatments and/or ongoing clinical trials and why?
- Can you direct me to any research that would give me confidence in the treatment(s) you propose for my kind of cancer?

- Is it better to get a second opinion now before anything is done, or wait till after the tests/surgery/other procedures that you may be recommending? Why?
- Do I have enough information? If not, what is lacking?

4. What are your specific recommendations?

- What are your reasons for recommending _____?
- Is there room for any flexibility?
- Can you point to research about the specific intervention(s) you are recommending for my kind of cancer?
- Where might I learn more about this method of treating my particular cancer?

5. The timing of treatment decisions and treatment

- Are the decisions I need to make taking shape in a timely fashion?
- What decisions must I make NOW: Who is recommending an immediate decision and why? If a physician is recommending immediate treatment within a few days, do I understand, and agree with, this urgency as a medical necessity? Is my condition life-threatening at this time? Have I had enough time to absorb the shock and make peace with my decision?
- What decisions can I make SOON: When? Who is recommending that I take time to come to a decision or that treatment is not necessary yet, and why? Do I understand, and agree with, this opportunity to take more time before embarking on treatment?
- What decisions can I make LATER: When? Who is recommending a later decision and why? Does a specific treatment have to come after or before another treatment?
- Do I need more information about any of the modalities before I can make my decision? If so, what and from whom?

- What amount of "wiggle-room" do I have to do further research, without being pressured by fear or time constraints?
- Do I know the time frame for any treatment suggested? And for recuperation?

6. What other concerns and general questions do I have?

- What is my prognosis? What is my life expectancy? Be truthful, please. (I understand that no one can predict exactly what any outcome will be.)
- Can you define remission? Is it disease free for, say, 5 years? How valid is that concept and what is it based on?
- What is the definition of "cure"? Does it mean disease-free for, say, 3–5 years, or for the rest of my life, or what?
- Is my cancer connected to any other kind of cancer? Is increased vigilance needed in any other part of my body?
- Do you have any suggestions of other things I could do to support my healing? Such as diet, etc?
- Can you recommend any research on acupuncture, massage, nutrition or other complementary modalities in relation to my type of cancer?
- I know you can't see into the future, but from your medical training what is the likely course of events if I do nothing?
- Does the hospital have a tissue bank? How long do they save the tissue and slides after a biopsy or surgery?

7. Questions for a surgeon (breast cancer)

- What is a "lumpectomy"? What does it remove—only the "cancer" cells? lymph nodes? sentinal nodes? If so, under what circumstances would you remove them?
- How large an area around the cancer will be cut out to ensure that all the cancer tissue is removed? (What will the margins be?)
- What is the statistical reoccurrence of cancer after a lumpectomy?

- How will my mobility be affected? How soon after surgery can I take part in sports and other activities?

- Are you recommending a lumpectomy because my body can't handle this itself? Is there another way to support my body to activate its own self-repairing system?

- You've mentioned following up with radiation: what would the radiation kill? What are the chances of damaging my heart/ my _____? What are the possible side effects? If radiation is recommended, why is it a necessary part of the treatment? If so, in my case, what are your reasons for suggesting radiation before, during, or after surgery?

- What do statistics show when comparing results with or without radiation? After five years? After ten years or longer? Likewise for estrogen blocking drugs (e.g. Tamoxifen), monoclonal anti-bodies and chemotherapy. (If you get easily depressed and discouraged with statistics, do not request statistical information.)

Regarding specific treatment interventions

8. Questions for a medical oncologist about chemotherapy and tests such as blood work

BEFORE CHEMOTHERAPY

- What chemotherapy drugs will be used? Name of drug? Potential side effects?

- How many treatments will I receive?

- How will I feel after each treatment?

- Will I need a port, shunt or catheter to receive the treatment? Please explain.

- Who will monitor my progress? How? Whom may I consult if I experience any problems with side effects?

- What will the long-term effects be?

- How will I know if the treatments are working?

- Can the cancer spread while I am being treated with chemotherapy?

- How can I tell if the cancer is coming back? Are there any danger signs to look out for?

- Are there any foods I should/should not take during treatment? What about alcohol? Smoking?
- Are there any exercises I should do or avoid during treatment?

DURING OR FOLLOWING CHEMOTHERAPY

- Can you tell me how I am progressing? Am I doing OK/better/worse than you might expect?
- List any problems you might be experiencing such as pain or side effects. Convey this to your oncologist, saying— for example:
  - The following things concern me: .
  - I am experiencing pain (describe) _____ in these areas _____. Is this normal during treatment? Why? What can I do to lessen it?
  - These are the medications I'm on _____. Will taking additional medication be safe/interfere with the ones I am already on?
  - I am experiencing these side effects _____. Is this normal during treatment? Why? What can I do to lessen them?

ABOUT BLOOD WORK

- Are you tracking a specific tumor marker in my case? If so, what is it? What is considered normal? What is mine? Are you satisfied with the results?
- How often will I have blood and tumor marker tests?
- What is my red blood count (HGB)? What is normal? How does mine compare with normal?
- What is my white blood count (WGB)? What is normal? How does mine compare with normal?

You are entitled to get copies of test results.

9. Questions before and after an MRI, X-ray, CT Scan or other tests

BEFORE

- Why are you suggesting this test?
- Who will administer this test, and where?

- Please describe what the procedure will entail? (Length of time, requirement to be immobile etc.)
- How soon will I get the results?
- Do I need to fast before this test? For how long?

AFTER
- Do the test results give you additional information? If so, what?
- Does it show improvement?
- If not, what is the next step? Do you recommend any other testing or a new treatment? If so, why?

10. Questions for a complementary or alternative (CAM) practitioner

Tell the practitioner clearly why you are seeking help—e.g. to complement your mainstream physicians, specifically for pain management or nausea, for a general consultation, or for an alternative approach, complete in itself. Then ask:

- What can I expect from your approach?
- How much experience have you had with cancer patients and specifically with my kind of cancer and my kind of mainstream treatments?
- Are you willing to work with mainstream doctors?
- What is the knowledge base for the treatment you are recommending? Specifically, are there any published data for this treatment?
- Are there any potential downsides?
- What is the length of treatment?
- If you are suggesting vitamins and supplements please specify brand names you know to be trustworthy and tell me why you are recommending them.
- How will your suggestions for diet, whole food and supplements affect my prescriptions for _____?
- What out-of-pocket costs will be involved? Fees for each visit? For supplements, etc?

OTHER PRIOR PREPARATION

- Mark all your appointments on a weekly or monthly calendar, noting time, place, and practitioner. Keep this calendar even *after* your appointments to verify your billing when it comes in.

- Find out well ahead of time whether you need to bring, mail or fax your medical history and any previous paper work or reports. Requirements often vary from office to office. Make the necessary arrangements to pick up your records from the originating office/hospital or have them forwarded in time for your appointment. If your doctor does not have your records in front of him, he may not be able to assess the situation properly.

- If your appointment is for a test, make sure you understand any pre-consultation instructions such as dietary restrictions.

ON THE DAY OF YOUR APPOINTMENT

- Meet the family member, friend or local oncology group representative who has agreed to accompany you early enough to share your list of questions and talk together about the purpose of your visit, and the kind of support you would appreciate.

- Call the office beforehand to find out if the doctor is on schedule, or whether an emergency has cropped up and your appointment will be delayed. This is not unusual, and you might be able to adjust your schedule accordingly.

- If you would like to record your visit, take along a small recording device, ready for that possibility.

- Think about how best to take care of yourself while waiting. For example, choose a good book, magazine or audio, a bottle of water—and a shawl for the cold examining rooms.

And be sure to bring your notebook with you.

At Appointments

IN THE WAITING ROOM OR FRONT OFFICE

- On arrival, be friendly to the person at the front desk, and make a note of his or her name. A receptionist can be a helpful ally when you are making future appointments or when you have practical questions to ask. Introduce your companion and indicate that you would like him/her to be present during the consultation.
- Relax with some deep breaths and feel your feet firmly on the ground.
- If a noisy TV is bothering you, ask if it's OK to turn the sound down or off. If the waiting room has no windows and little sign of ventilation, ask how long the wait will be. Perhaps you'll be able to take a short ten minute walk. If you find that the receptionist expects the doctor to be delayed, adjust the time of your walk or wait in your car in the parking lot, the hospital cafeteria or a local cafe. Check back just before the anticipated adjusted time or, before you leave the waiting room, request that the receptionist call your cell phone when the health professional is almost ready to see you.
- Ask the person accompanying you to be prepared to take notes for you and remind him or her of what you particularly wish the focus to be.
- Add any last minute questions to your list that arise while you are waiting.

IN THE CONSULTING ROOM—INITIAL CONNECTIONS AND QUESTIONS

- If your anxiety level is high when entering the office, remind yourself that the person accompanying you is there to support you. Even if you don't always hear or remember everything that is being said, your companion will catch things you might miss. Keep breathing *and* stay present.
- Ask the physician for permission to record the consultation, if you wish to do so.
- Listen to what the doctor has to say. Note any questions that arise while you are listening and check off those that

have been addressed. Ask for clarification whenever you feel you need it.

- Go through your list of questions and ask all of them systematically.

- If you feel rushed, breathe deeply again and ask the health practitioner to slow down. Ask your companion if she/he understands the gist of what is being said, and to rephrase the answer back to you to make sure you understand it.

- Feeling that you are interviewing your doctor may also boost your confidence. Your questions are NOT an imposition on your health providers. Questions help practitioners to know more about you, so that they can do a better job.

- If your physician doesn't appear be listening to you or is not willing to answer your questions, that person may not be the best professional for you.

Your questions are NOT an imposition on your health providers. Questions help practitioners to know more about you, so that they can do a better job.

- Do *not* sign up for treatment on the spot. You need time to integrate what you have heard before you come to a decision.

IN THE CONSULTING ROOM—TALKING TO A DOCTOR ABOUT SIDE EFFECTS OF CANCER AND ITS TREATMENTS

1. ABOUT PAIN

You need not be stoical about pain. There are many ways to find relief including medication, acupuncture, meditation, prayer, relaxation, yoga, hypnosis, guided imagery, application of heat or cold, exercise, massage and energy work. These methods are not mutually exclusive.

- Note the things you do that help to alleviate pain. Note anything that increases it.

- If you need prescription medication for the pain, be sure to tell your doctor the exact location of the pain and give a clear description of your symptoms, and any other medication you are taking.

- You may be asked to rate your pain on a scale of 0-5, (0 = least, 5 = most). Sometimes a scale of 0-10 is used.

- Note when the pain started and where it is located. Use descriptive words, such as achy, sharp, tight, gnawing, pulsing, numbing, tingling, dull, tender, throbbing, radiating, cold, hot, shooting, intense, nagging, blinding, nauseating, unbearable, etc.

- If pain medication isn't working sufficiently or if you have side effects, contact your doctor again, explain the medication you are on, the treatment you are following and describe your symptoms as above.

2. About Sexual Issues

If you fear that illness or treatment will bring losses of attractiveness, sexual desire, sexual functioning, or fertility, talk with your doctor. Many cancer treatments do bring fatigue, nausea, pain and weakness, none of which is conducive to good sex. However, in the last twenty years, important advances have been made in treating these problems.

- Before you agree to any treatment, discuss your sexual concerns with your physician or the person in your health care team with whom you feel most trust and most relaxed.

- Ask that professional about changes affecting sexuality that may occur due to cancer treatments and medication. This will help you make more informed treatment decisions and prepare for possible outcomes. If you do experience changes, ask about help available.

- Share your concerns with your partner and discover how to enjoy sensuous pleasures together.

- Gradually build up your physical vitality through exercise, walking, swimming or other activities that will help increase your energy, flexibility and strength. Start slowly, e.g. walking instead of jogging.

3. SHARING YOUR CONCERNS ABOUT OTHER SIDE EFFECTS

Before, or in addition to, consulting your doctor, review and try out these tips from practitioners and patients about fatigue, infection, nausea, hair loss, memory loss, mouth sores, fluid retention, lymphedema or neuropathy:

Fatigue

Fatigue is a common symptom of cancer itself and its treatments.

- Rest often, take naps and go to bed early.
- Drink lots of water to eliminate waste from your body.
- Go for short walks.
- Don't overdo it when you are feeling well. Pace yourself.
- Delegate chores to others, but do something enjoyable for yourself.

Infection and depletion of your immune system

- Wash your hands frequently.
- Avoid anyone with a cold, flu or infection.
- Avoid all dental work, even cleaning, during chemotherapy.
- Try not to break your skin—use a soft toothbrush, don't cut or tear your cuticles or scratch pimples, and do use gloves during housework. If you have dry skin, use lotions and pat yourself dry.
- Avoid contact with all animal litter boxes or birdcages.

Nausea

- Eat small meals frequently, but slowly, chewing each bite well.
- Drink liquids slowly 30-60 minutes after a meal.
- Avoid strong smelling, spicy, fatty, sweet or fried foods.
- If you feel sick in the morning, eat crackers or dry toast before getting out of bed.
- Make a list of foods that are easy for you to eat. Miso soups and broths? Oatmeal? Mashed potatoes? Cooked veggies? Fruit juices? Eggs? Ginger tea?

Hair loss (alopecia)

Chemotherapy often causes hair loss. Before you undergo chemotherapy:

- Have your hair cut in a short style.
- Use a mild shampoo and a soft hairbrush. Don't pull hard when combing.
- Sleep on a satin pillow.

If you do lose your hair:

- Try on a free wig from your local cancer group.
- Cover your head while in the sun.

Mouth sores (oral mucositis)

Because the lining of your mouth is very delicate, its cells can often be affected by chemotherapy. To help prevent mouth sores:

- Have your teeth cleaned, and any oral infections treated, prior to chemo.
- Brush twice a day with a soft brush and floss gently once a day.
- Don't use a harsh mouthwash. Instead try rinsing four times per day with 1 teaspoon each of salt and baking soda dissolved in a pint of water. It's important to keep bacteria under control.
- Avoid rough foods, which scrape the inside of your mouth such as crusty breads.
- Ice chips and popsicles can ease pain. Talk to your doctor about other solutions.

Fluid retention, lymphedema and neuropathy

- To ease fluid retention, avoid table salt and high sodium foods and try a diuretic tea. You can consult your doctor if you still have this problem.
- Lymphedema, swelling in the arms or legs as a result of blocked lymphatic vessels, can occur after surgery. Lymph massage from a trained practitioner and compression arm or leg stockings can be helpful.
- Peripheral neuropathy, tingling or numbness, is sometimes caused by anti-cancer drugs that affect the nerves going to

the fingers and toes. Some herbs and supplements may be helpful (e.g. yerba mate tea). Consult a naturopath.

Memory loss

"Chemo-brain" is not a figment of your imagination. Many people experience memory problems and "fuzzy" thinking after undergoing chemotherapy. These effects can emerge many months later.

- "Chemo-brain" is an active area of research, but definitive solutions have yet to be found.
- Consult a naturopath for natural supplements.

Appetite loss

There may be times when your loss of appetite is troubling to yourself and others. If you do not *look* sick, it is sometimes difficult for your loved ones not to push food on you.

- It is better to have food available that you like to nibble, when you do feel like eating, rather than forcing a "proper" meal down your throat when you don't feel up to it.
- Ask your practitioner to suggest some easily digestible foods.

Immediately After Each Appointment

WHILE YOUR MEMORY IS STILL FRESH

- *As soon after your appointment as possible*, review with your companion what was said and the course of action suggested by the professional. Details can fade very fast.

- Refer to your notes especially if you did not record the appointment and underline the important points—regarding your diagnosis, answers to your questions, and recommendations. If you are not sure about any aspect of the discussion or if your perceptions differ greatly from those of the person accompanying you, identify the area of confusion and reframe questions to clarify it.

- Consider faxing your questions to your doctor's office for attention.

- If you come away from an appointment sensing your questions were not being addressed, or you are not clear about an explanation, don't consider your lack of understanding as unintelligent or your doubts as silly. Honor them as contributing to your well-being—and note questions you now wish to ask. If necessary, talk to someone from an oncology support group who understands medical implications.

- **Use the *Following up a Visit* exploration on the next page** when you get home. It provides a framework to make record keeping easy after each practitioner (mainstream or complementary) or hospital appointment.

  - ~ Clearly identify each meeting with the medical professional's name and the date at the top of the page and place that page in your three-ring notebook or file.

  - ~ Note any matters that you want to follow-up—further research, reading, or interviews. Include your personal observations and impressions. Add self-care (non-medical) ideas that you might also wish to explore.

- If your writing is very difficult to read, consider typing, or ask someone to type key information.

If you come away from an appointment sensing your questions were not being addressed, or you are not clear about an explanation, don't consider your lack of understanding unintelligent or your doubts silly.

Following up a visit

Record your answers to the questions below that are important to you after each healthcare appointment.

Date _____

Name of Med. Professional _____

Reason for Visit _____

Diagnosis given _____

Test(s) used, if any _____

Review the list of questions you took with you and the notes you or your companion made during or just after the meeting. To help you clarify your thoughts and feelings, ask yourself if all your questions answered.

• If so, highlight or outline briefly the important information. Then place these notes in a place ready for filing for when you develop your system for organizing your papers. (See Chapters 5 and 6)

• If not, ask yourself (and make notes accordingly):
  ~ Which questions still require an answer?
  ~ Are there any technical/medical words that I don't fully understand?

Health professional's recommendations

• List immediate recommendations:

• List "down the line" recommendations:

• What are my thoughts and feelings about each of these recommendations?

Personal impressions of the practitioner, the staff and the facility

• What strengths and/or weakness did I observe/experience during this visit?

• How does my experience at this appointment affect my willingness to continue with this professional?

• Other thoughts and gut reactions?

Follow-up actions

- Schedule an additional test?
- Get a second opinion/see another practitioner?
- Schedule recommended treatment?
- Explore further research?
- Check out other resources recommended?
- What decisions are wise to postpone until I have further information or additional test results?

After every visit update your medical history

Keep a chronological log of all your treatments as outlined in Item 2 of *Appendix I Build Your Own Yellow Pages*. It will become a useful reference for all your practitioners, as well as for yourself.

Make a note of your next appointment in your calendar.

SUN	MON	TUES	WED	THURS	FRI	SAT

After a Series of Appointments

From time to time it's wise to review your progress and renew your commitment to good health. Remember, your health is in your hands as well as your doctor's.

Reviewing your medical healthcare progress

Use the suggestions in this worksheet to review your medical healthcare progress at regular intervals after a number of visits—weekly, monthly or whenever you wish to take an inventory. This will help you to get an overview of a bigger picture and notice if anything is falling through the cracks.

FOR THE PERIOD FROM _____ TO _____

1. **What appointments have been most important to me?**

2. **What are the most significant ideas to have emerged from conversations?**

   For each note:

   • Date _____

   • With whom?_____

   • About?_____

   • How might I follow-up these ideas and leads? _____

3. **Progress**

• Is there an overall treatment plan in place?

   ~ If not, who can help me put one in place?

   ~ If so, how is this plan progressing? What specific progress has been made on previous decisions or since my last review?

• Is my treatment plan proceeding in a timely manner?

   ~ Do I feel rushed to make decisions?

   ~ Do I feel impatient about the slow rate of progress?

4. Communication

- Am I being kept informed? Am I sufficiently included in the decision-making loop?
  - ~ Have reports been sent to the practitioners I have so requested?
  - ~ Are my health care providers communicating about, and coordinating, my treatment? If not, where specifically is coordination lacking?

5. Treatment Goals

- What are my treatment goals?
  - ~ For next week?
  - ~ Next month?
  - ~ Three months hence?

6. Other observations

- How do I feel?
- How is my body responding to treatment?
- Am I experiencing any differences in my sleep pattern? Or any fatigue, aches, pains or unusual body sensations?

Check often that your treatment log is fully up-to-date and that you have noted all upcoming appointments in your calendar.

Reviewing your personal progress

Can you say "yes" to the following statements?

1. I am eliminating as much stress as possible.

2. I have confidence in my doctors and in my treatment.

3. I am keeping the scheduled appointments and treatments that I have committed to.

4. I will persevere even when things are difficult.

5. I believe I will be among those who survive my kind of cancer.

6. I am now ready to make changes in my lifestyle to increase my chances of wellness, for example:

    • I am willing to exercise/walk/or _____

    • I am willing to limit/give up my intake of alcohol, tobacco, sugar, or _____

    • I am also choosing to change_____

This could also be a good time to reread personal notes if you keep a journal. If you are doing your best, congratulate yourself—and keep going.

Take this book, your notes and questions to your visits.

**Your cancer care can be
a well-coordinated experience.**

Keep Your Sanity— Organize the Paper Trail

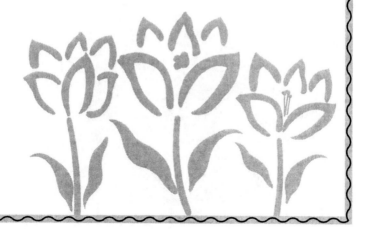

5

Keep it Simple—
A Preliminary Approach
to Getting Organized

A S YOUR RECORDS AND NOTES ACCUMULATE, THEY WILL become your personal collection of information— tidbits from conversations, questions for your surgeon, notes on conversations with your physician or health provider, as well as official reports ranging from lab work and X-rays to insurance coverage and hospital bills; from medical releases to privacy statements; from the latest research on the treatment of your particular cancer to newsletters of local cancer support groups.

When initially diagnosed, I was blissfully unaware of the need to organize the papers connected to my cancer. But suddenly, overnight it seemed, my paperwork and handwritten jottings became so unmanageable that I couldn't find specific information when I needed it.

DISORGANIZATION IS HAZARDOUS TO YOUR HEALTH!

Unnecessary distractions from disorganized record keeping will dissipate and drain your energy—the very energy you need for healing. The more doctors' visits, the more you will require a system to separate out different types of information. You may find yourself facing many a frustrating moment as you try to understand and organize the paperwork.

There are many ways to divide your paperwork. The kind of preliminary sorting of papers and notes suggested in this chapter may work quite well for you, especially if you tend to resist organization and want to take it easy. Or, you may prefer the more detailed choices in Chapter 6. Whatever system you choose, adapt it according to your own needs.

Guidelines to Keep it Simple

Step 1: GET THE SUPPLIES YOU WILL NEED

- 8½" x11" three ring binder (1½" thick or bigger) and paper
- Post-it sticky notes, and/or binder dividers with tabs
- Paperclips and/or a stapler
- Three hole-punch
- Folders or file boxes

Step 2: GATHER YOUR PAPERWORK

- Gather all the paperwork connected with your cancer journey, including notes, newsletters and magazines.
- Clear and reserve a space on a bookshelf for books, and other relevant material.

Step 3: SORT IT OUT

- Put bulky items, such as articles and newsletters, that will not fit in a binder, into folders or file boxes, and place them on your shelf.
- Spread all the remaining loose papers out on the top of a table or on the floor so you can easily see what you have.
- Discard duplicates and illegible or unnecessary papers.
- Sort the papers into groups of similar items in whatever way suits you intuitively. Examples might be:
  - ~ Notes from conversations with friends
  - ~ Questions for my physicians and their answers
  - ~ Test results
  - ~ Ideas to follow up
  - ~ Bills, insurance letters… and so on.
- Clip the papers of each group together.
- Identify each group by writing its name on a Post-it sticker or a brightly colored slip of paper and put that on the front page of each group.
- Re-order the papers within each group in whatever way makes sense to you, for example, by date or by service provided.

Step 4: Insert Your Papers Into An 8 1/2 X 11" Three-ring Binder

- Punch holes in your papers.
- Insert each group of papers into your binder/loose-leaf notebook in whatever order you have chosen.
- If you wish, create sections by naming and adding tabbed dividers.

Step 5: Build Your Own *Yellow Pages*

Turn to *Appendix I: Build Your Own Yellow Pages*. This provides an easy structure within which to compile a record of all your most important cancer-related contacts and frequently used resources—a ready reference directory at your fingertips.

- **Create and fill out** *Yellow Pages* **1 and 2** (on paper of your choice).

  Page 1. Your Most-Frequently-Used Telephone/ Email Contacts & Emergency Numbers

  Make a list of the contact information you expect to refer to constantly. Knowing exactly where to turn for a particular phone number can prevent a lot of unnecessary stress.

  Page 2. Your Chronological Cancer Log

  Follow the suggestions given to track your cancer journey from first symptoms (if any) and discovery of your cancer, through diagnosis, follow-up tests and results, treatment decisions and all appointments. Keep this record of your progress up-to-date. You can refer to it during an office visit.

- Place a copy of these completed Pages 1 and 2 in the front of your binder, OR put them in a section named *My Yellow Pages*, wherever you can reach for them automatically without thinking, so that they are easily accessible at all times.

Pages 1 and 2 are now ready to take to all professional visits. You will not have to rack your brain to remember details, and it may prevent you from blanking out, when physicians ask for such information.

What matters is that you know where to find everything —at the drop of a hat!

Fill out the remaining *Yellow Pages* 3–13 (on paper of your choice):

> Page 3. Personal Contacts
>
> Page 4. Mainstream Medical Health Professionals
>
> Page 5. Complementary Health Professionals
>
> Page 6. Labs and Other Facilities Giving Reports
>
> Page 7. Pharmacies & Medications; Vitamins, Minerals and Supplements
>
> Page 8. Health Insurance, Legal & Financial Contacts
>
> Page 9. Possible Leads
>
> Page 10. Favorite or Most Frequently-Used Resources
>
> Page 11. How Others Can Help
>
> Page 12. Thank You List
>
> Page 13. Where to Find It

- Place them in *My Yellow Pages* in your binder.
- Make sure you continually update these pages.

With these six steps, you have in hand a simple system to enable you to find information when you need it and to incorporate new paperwork as it accumulates.

Step 6: ORGANIZE PAPERS FOR SPECIFIC MEDICAL APPOINTMENTS

Create a "traveling" binder, with a heading such as *"For My Next Visit,"* by changing the contents according to the purpose of each visit:

- At the front, keep a copy of your updated *Yellow Pages 1 and 2.*

Before each visit

- Ask "What papers do I need to take with me?"
- Transfer information such as previous tests and reports, and a list of questions for the practitioner to your "traveling binder." For a second opinion consultation, it is likely that you will need most, or all, of your medical information. For follow-up visits with your regular doctor you will need much less.

After each visit return the papers you have transferred back to their original location.

Puja

**What I Did
Initially**

From the start, I put a list of frequently used telephone numbers right at the front of my binder.

Then I made three piles—1) medical papers, 2) papers connected with my support team and 3) information about cancer. I sub-divided each pile: I divided my medical information according to each professional. I put everything connected with doctor 'A' together and everything connected with doctor 'B' together—letters, prescriptions for medication and tests, test results, notes, billing etc. I rearranged each pile in dated order with the most recent papers in front of earlier ones. I wrote the practitioner's name on a brightly colored slip of paper and attached it to the topmost current page. After punching the holes, I placed the pages for each practitioner in alphabetical order in my binder.

I divided up everything connected to my personal support team according to each individual, group or organization and arranged each set separately alphabetically.

When it came to sorting cancer resources, I found that people had given me articles, newsletters and magazines that were too big or too awkward a size to fit in a binder, yet too floppy to stand easily by themselves on my bookshelf. I improvised by placing them in folders and then I put them together in a file box.

Tory

**Learning to
Keep Track**

You'd be surprised what you can forget! I couldn't imagine forgetting the dates of such momentous events like surgeries, treatments and tests. I thought they were indelibly etched on my brain.

Now, twelve years after my initial diagnosis, it's almost impossible to remember even approximate dates, past or recent. I have looked blank so many times when a doctor has asked me, "When was ___?" or "When did you___?" that I have finally started a log of all visits and tests.

**What matters is that you know where you can find
everything—at the drop of a hat!**

For a more detailed and comprehensive approach, read on. The next chapter provides numerous hints and suggestions to help you deal with specific types of paperwork and the people connected to them. Divide and Conquer!

6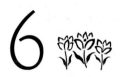

Divide and Conquer!
A More Comprehensive
System of Organization

A S THE NUMBER OF PAPERS INCREASE, YOU MAY WANT TO organize further. Here are additional guidelines for tracking and dealing with the multitude of paperwork and reports connected to practitioners, finance, insurance, legal records, cancer information and personal notes. Before you proceed to Step 7, make sure you've completed Steps 1 through 6 in Chapter 5.

You may find that you now need either additional binders or one that is much thicker.

Step 7: CREATE SEVEN SECTIONS FOR YOUR BINDER(S)

You will need more dividers, with tabs both large and small. Divide your papers into the following categories, naming a divider with a LARGE tab for each:

Section 1: Practitioners For papers from doctors and health-related practitioners (and their staff).

Section 2: Reports/Tests For medical reports & results.

Section 3: Finance/Insurance For financial, billing, insurance, money, and tax issues.

Section 4: Legal For legal papers, both current (e.g. medical releases and privacy statements) as well as about the future (e.g. health care proxy and living will).

Section 5: Info/Resources For information about cancer, including articles, magazines and websites.

Section 6: Personal For everything that supports you personally—contacts, writing etc.

Section 7: My *Yellow Pages*

Some helpful tips:

- **As you organize Sections 1 and 2,** refer to Chapters 3 and 4 for hints for dealing with professional support and appointments.

- **As you organize Sections 3 and 4**, note the numerous suggestions for billing, finance and insurance, legal, tax *and* personnel matters within this chapter. These topics are NOT covered elsewhere in the text.

- **As you organize Sections 5**, refer to the many resources in *Appendix 2* and the chapter endnotes.

- **As you organize Section 6**, refer to Chapter 2.

Section 1: Paperwork From Your Health-related Practitioners

You may be surprised at the number of mainstream doctors you will be asked to consult, and in addition you may have complementary care appointments. It is best to keep each separate.

Identify all your currently *active* practitioners

- Put the name/role of each on a divider with a SMALL tab.
- Arrange these dividers in alphabetical order behind the larger tab for Practitioners
  - ~ If, for example, your active team includes your primary care physician, healer, oncologist, nutritionist, radiologist, and surgeon, you would have six subdivisions, one for each.[1]
  - ~ You don't need to make a tab for everyone in an office. (i.e. All paperwork with regard to primary care physician, his or her nurse, physician's assistant, and receptionist would go together behind one tab.)

How to organize your practitioners' paper trail

- Organize each practitioner's papers in dated order (most recent on top or in whatever way works for you): Include records of all consultations or visits, your preparatory questions, doctors' answers, your follow-up notes, and prescriptions or recommendations you receive.
  - ~ Clip or staple.
  - ~ Three-hole punch.
  - ~ Place behind the appropriate dividers.
- Add dividers and tabs for other professionals as they become active in your treatment.
- Add your notes regarding your choice of care and your professional visits as per Chapters 3 and 4.

Note: Do not include financial or legal papers along with your medical papers. It is more efficient to keep them in a separate section.

Section 2: Medical Reports and Test Results

Health-related reports will come in a variety of shapes and sizes from many sources such as hospital departments and laboratories. In the beginning it may not seem necessary to separate the reports but later it becomes essential as more and more information will come your way.

How to keep track of your medical reports

Identify tests you have had such as blood work, lab results, pathology and consultation records and ask your doctor or hospital to provide copies of results.

- Put the name of each type of test on a small tab divider. [2]
  - ~ Arrange dividers in alphabetical order behind the Reports/Results divider.
  - ~ Put the medical reports and test results from each type of test together, in dated order, behind these dividers. For example, keep radiology reports and blood work reports separate from each other within this section. It will then be easier to reference them at your next visit or set of tests.

~ Highlight the date of test results or lab-work.

- Add notes you have made related to going for tests and receiving results.
- Keep medical release forms and privacy statements connected to these tests in Section 4: Legal records.

If you are asked by one doctor for reports or slides from another doctor, if at all possible, arrange to pick them up and carry them there yourself, unless an internal system, say, between a doctor and a hospital already exists.

Section 3: Financial, Billing and Insurance Records

It is wise to keep your financial and insurance records in a third section of the binder. **Do not mix them with other medical notes** pertaining to health practitioners or test results. Consider keeping them in a separate second binder—especially if you already have a lot of medical information. This is information you are unlikely to want to carry to your appointments.

Health providers and insurance companies are closely connected through billing practices so, if you have health insurance, keep doctors' bills together with insurance bills.

How to track billing and insurance payments

Before you file anything connected to billing and insurance, review it very carefully:

- If it is urgent, put it in a special folder earmarked for that purpose with a name such as "IMMEDIATE ATTENTION," and keep it in an obvious place where you cannot forget it. Then take action as soon as you can.
- Put the bills that do *not* need to be paid immediately in a folder named "BILLS" until you know how you will deal with them.
- Review this folder once per week; specifically, divide the bills into 2 main categories, *non-reimbursable* and *reimbursable* bills, and file them according to the following guidelines.

1. NON-REIMBURSABLE BILLS—You alone are responsible for paying these bills.

Divide non-reimbursable billing into the following two sections, naming a *small* tab for each:

- *Non-reimbursable—Bills pending*
  Use this section until a bill has been paid and is acknowledged as paid.
- *Non-reimbursable—Bills paid*
  Use this section when no further payment is required in connection with the charge.

2. REIMBURSABLE BILLS—Bills you expect your insurance company to pay in part or in whole.

Divide reimbursable billing into three sections and again prepare divider tabs to identify each:

- *Reimbursable—Bills Pending*
  Use this section for all bills you receive until they have been paid and acknowledged as by paid by all concerned.
- *Reimbursable—Bills Paid by Primary Insurance*
  File here only those bills that require *no* further payment in connection with the charge.

- *Reimbursable—Bills Paid by Secondary Insurance* (if any)
  Likewise file when it is clear that no further payment is required in connection with the charge.

It is especially important to separate out bills pending from bills paid if you and your insurance are each paying a portion.

ABOUT BILLS

Check thoroughly before you pay any bill. Bills often arrive quite a long time after your actual appointment, and may have a name on it that you find hard to recognize. I found I had to look at each bill more than once. Refer to your medical calendar to check that the date on the bill corresponds to the date of the appointment.

Sometimes statements are very confusing. You may receive a bill that looks as if a hospital expects you to pay, but it is actually the insurance company's responsibility. In addition, instructions regarding payment may be very confusing.

Once, on the front of a bill, large bold print announced, **"Please detach and return this portion with your payment."** When I couldn't understand why this had not been sent to my insurance company, I asked a friend to help me. She pointed out the small light italic script I had overlooked, *"Please read the back of this statement."* On the reverse side were instructions to attach a copy of my insurance card, if valid. Statements that look like bills can easily fool you and, if you don't get help, you might mail a check unnecessarily.

You are not stupid. Some billing is just plain tricky. Sometimes persistence is needed.

- Before paying a bill, make a copy of the bill and file it. Note on the bill the date on which you paid it, the check number, and the name of any person you spoke to in connection with the payment.

- Ask if the hospital has a patient's guide to billing. Such a guide can be helpful if you are not familiar with that hospital's billing practices.

- Ask for help if you are not confident about interpreting bills—I found it was better to ask before I landed in a muddle. If friends or family members can't offer this type of help, contact the person in the billing department of your physician's office, or a social worker.

- Keep copies of all medical bills, insurance statements (often called Explanation of Benefits or EOB's) and receipts in order to check for accuracy. This will serve you well when it's tax time.

- Online tracking of bills is now quite common—most insurance companies now have online portals where customers can register to track their records.

BE ALERT WHEN YOUR BILLS COME IN

Miriam shares how she learned to pay attention to her bills: When she was fully involved in her initial treatment, Miriam just stashed bills in a folder for later attention. Ignoring them didn't make them go away and it took her months to get that pile of bills taken care of. She discovered she needed to maintain a clear record of the date of every appointment in order to match it up to the billing when it came in—sometimes months later—as in these examples:

Miriam In July 2004 I had a biopsy, which led me to know that my lump was malignant. Well into my treatment, eleven months later, in June the following year, I got a lab bill from the hospital for $33.75. I didn't send it in—I figured my insurance would cover it and I never heard from them again until October 2005: but the bill was not from the hospital. It was from a collection agency telling me I owed them $33.75!! One bill and there it was—sent for collection. Although I don't know what happened, I think that the hospital had misfiled the claim with my insurance company as I do have a $15 co-pay. I just sent in the money and told them how ridiculous it was. I learned I could not rely on my health care providers in doctors' offices, labs or hospitals to file claims accurately. Even though the instructions on insurance forms are clear, they didn't always send it to the proper address provided. In fact I often had to call them or my insurance company to get bills straightened out. It seems we really have to fight for the coverage that is in our policy.

Two weeks after my surgery, my physician asked me if I would I like to hear about a new type of radiation—and since the doctor who was working with the clinical trials just happened to be there that day, I agreed. This doctor explained it to me (for less than ten minutes) but I decided I was not interested in pursuing it. Nine months later I received a bill for $250 for the conversation! I could not believe it! Technically she was asking me to participate in a clinical trial and yet she was charging me to hear about it. This time I did not pay. I wrote a searing letter to them and never heard from them again. Hopefully your experience will not be as bad as mine. We certainly need to stay alert.

Put your own system into place, take nothing for granted, stay on top of it, and always ask for help when you need it.

About Insurance Coverage

Before you get any treatment, review your policy. It is prudent to know the answers to these questions:

• What are my outpatient benefits?

• What are my inpatient benefits?

• Does my insurance company cover out-of-network as well as in-network providers?

• What is my annual deductible? When does my policy renew?

- What are the co-payments or percentage co-insurance I have to make for each?
- How do I file a claim?
- Will my insurance cover second opinions? Clinical trials? Home health care? Etc
- When **must** I get preauthorization for treatment or consultations?

As soon as you are able, find the answers to these questions since annual deductibles, co-payments per office visit, test, prescription drugs (brand name and generic), ambulance service, or wellness care allowed can vary greatly. Even if you have the same insurance and you renew your plan, contact your insurance company at the beginning of the year to review your benefits for any changes.

Many different types of health plans exist, including group plans, individual plans, HMOs (health maintenance organization), PPOs (preferred provider organization), disability income insurance, long-term care plans and Medicaid, and for seniors—Medicare. There are now specific personal *cancer* indemnity plans in some states.

Because of the Affordable Care Act (ACA) and the increased complexity of health care insurance, for example the advent of HSAs (health savings account), HRAs (health reimbursement arrangement), FSAs (flexible spending account), and MSAs (medical savings account), it is difficult to be too specific about how to navigate these systems or to know what changes may be made in the future. Make sure you understand your health care plan and its benefits. Meet with a representative if needed, so that you are clear about your coverage.

The right kind of coverage should provide benefits for inpatient hospital care, physician services, lab work and X-rays, prescription drugs, outpatient services and nursing home care at a location of your choice. If necessary, get help from your insurance provider to understand it.

- If pre-authorization for a specific treatment is required, find out who has to make the treatment referral.
- Enter your insurance information including membership I.D., plan name and policy numbers for all your insurance carriers, in your *Yellow Pages*.

Submitting claims

Expect health care providers to make a copy of your current insurance card(s) at your first visit and to submit a claim on your behalf. Make sure this is the case. If not, then you will have to handle this yourself. If you don't receive your EOB (explanation of benefit)—in a timely fashion, check in with them to make sure they have followed through.

When I pursued an allowable claim through the billing department of my surgeon's office, the staff was most helpful, and the insurance company backed down on their previous rejection.

If necessary, get help filing claims. Again, if friends can't help, a local Legal Aid office, Office of Aging or hospital social service department might be able to put you in touch with a person specifically paid to do this. Your state might also have advocates in their health or banking and insurance departments.

Better still, some insurance companies have case managers. In a situation where you are likely to have on-going contact with your insurer, ask if they will assign a case manager to you. That's not always possible, so if you find yourself talking to a particularly helpful representative, thank that person, request his or her name and telephone extension, and ask to be connected to that extension in future calls.

If you don't understand a bill or an Explanation of Benefits or if the amount is different from what you expect, keep asking questions. Insurance companies can make mistakes. Be persistent. If you have Medicare coverage, you might find answers to your questions online at www.medicare.gov

If your insurance company rejects a claim that has been submitted, call the company to ask their representative why it was rejected. Then immediately call the billing person in your medical professional's office. Explain what the insurance representative told you and ask them to look into the matter on your behalf. If you are still not satisfied, don't give up—file again.

A wrong code for your diagnosis is a common error. Other reasons a claim is denied include a decision that your procedure was not medically necessary, that you have a pre-exisiting condition or that you have chosen to go "out-of-network."

If a claim you still understand to be justified is again rejected, request the insurance company's appeal process and make an appeal. Ask someone to review your letter before you send it in to make sure it is clear and accurate.

If you feel that the insurance company is inappropriately handling your case, or if you have a continuing unresolved dispute, lodge a complaint with your state's Insurance Department. You may be able to do this online. A local Legal Aid office might also help.

- Keep a written record of all calls you make, noting:

    Date _____

    Time _____

    Person who spoke to you _____

    Claim number _____

    Question, issue or dispute discussed _____

    Answer/action needed _____

- Keep a written record of all correspondence with your insurance company, claim forms and copies of bills.
- **Don't get discouraged**. Take a break, go for a walk, have a cup of tea, call up a friend, ask for help and come back to it later.

For Those with Financial Difficulties

If you have worries about health care costs and/or still do not have insurance coverage, speak to your physician, a medical social worker, a social services department or the business office of the hospital or clinic about financial assistance. You may be eligible for services provided by volunteer or not-for-profit organizations, especially if you are low-income, under- or uninsured.

Community agencies and religious service organizations such as the Salvation Army, Catholic Charities, and Jewish Social Services, may be able to help. Some organizations exist to benefit a specific population such as children, women, seniors or those with a specific kind of cancer. Your local librarian may be a valuable resource for information.

Many pharmaceutical manufacturers offer drug reimbursement costs or patient assistance programs to those who are not eligible for Medicare or Medicaid and who do not have private insurance to help pay for costs of their drugs used in treatment.

- Don't spend money unnecessarily—especially on incidentals. Even though a well-intentioned spouse or partner says, "Don't worry now, we'll pay later," consider if an expenditure is really necessary. Expenses do mount up. For example, you may not always need to buy an expensive brand name, say, of a body lotion or cream. Ask your doctor if you can use cream you already have at home.

- Don't write off the generosity of friends. In a truly difficult financial crisis, a fundraising activity may allow friends and family to open their hearts and their wallets.

ABOUT TAX DEDUCTIONS

Create a sub-section for other financial papers related to your illness such as material from your tax-preparer, financial advisor, or other business professionals.

- Ask a tax-preparer or financial adviser about tax deductions in connection with your illness.

- Keep an accurate record of all your medical expenses for the IRS. Note mileage and keep all gas, toll, hotel, meal, rail, bus and airline receipts for every health related journey as well as other out-of-pocket expenses such as prescription drugs and medical equipment. The records will be needed when you claim them as part of your medical tax deductions at the end of the financial year.

- When you are claiming medical deductions, make a year-end tally of all your expenses as follows:

Total premium payments	$ _____
Total travel expenses	$ _____
Total co-pay	$ _____
Total co-insurance	$ _____
Total prescriptions	$ _____
Total	**$** _____

- Subtract any payments reimbursed by your insurance company, as you will not be able to claim them.

Section 4: Legal Records

It is practical to divide your legal records according to *current* treatment and *future* life choices.

Current treatment—create sub-sections with smaller tabs for each of the following:

- Consent forms for treatment
- Medical release forms
- Privacy statements

Future life choices—create sub-sections with smaller tabs for your lawyer or for each of your advanced directives:

- Living Will
- Health Proxy (Health care power of attorney)
- Will & Power of Attorney
- Ethical will

Consider getting a fire-proof box for important papers.

How to organize your legal records

ABOUT YOUR CURRENT TREATMENT AND THE LAW

What has the law got to do with medical treatment? A lot!

Signing forms

You will find yourself signing forms before you see a doctor or get medical treatment. These include documents giving permission for tests or treatment to begin, permission for your records to be released from one doctor to another, and hospital/medical office privacy statements.

Before you sign up for treatment it is your right to know from your doctor exactly what is entailed, including any risks, in terms you can understand, so you can compare risks to expected benefits.

- **DO NOT SIGN any consent forms, if the exact procedure has not been described or if you do not understand it. Your consent must be fully informed.**

- Cross out statements that are not in agreement with your wishes. Even if your doctor has forceful opinions and strong recommendations, it is your decision and responsibility, as a mentally competent adult, to accept or refuse treatment.

Your rights: privacy statements & other concerns

You do have a number of rights. For example, you generally have the right to inspect and ask for a copy of your records, to amend your records if you find inaccurate or incorrect information, to identify others who have received your information, and to request confidential communications.

Since signing privacy forms seem to me to benefit institutions, not patients, sometimes I noted beside my name, "I am signing to indicate that I have read the privacy statement—not that I am in agreement."

When it comes to those privacy statements that all patients are now asked to sign, you are signing a mandated disclosure form, not a contract. It is merely a record that proves that you were informed in writing as to how your information will be used and shared. Refusing to sign will not change the offices' ability to share your information.

In fact, if a national system of electronic medical records is put in place, as some hope, shared medical information could save your life. But there is a trade-off: the security of your personal health information could be at stake. For example, your personal information could be used "for training," and demographic information and the dates that you received treatment might be used for fund-raiser activities supported by your hospital or doctor's office.[3]

Since The Health Insurance Portability and Accountability Act (HIPAA), currently does not give you the right to opt out in most cases, and the agreements can change at any time, think about the personal information you have given your doctor in good faith.

- If you have given your doctor any very personal or embarrassing information, ask if he or she would be willing to keep it out of your record as long as its absence would not negatively affect the quality of your care or your health.

- If you do not understand what you are signing, be sure to ask questions.

Work related issues

If you find it necessary to take time off from employment, check out the following support to help you negotiate the best arrangements. There are disability laws to protect you, specifically two federal acts:

- The Americans with Disabilities Act (ADA) requires employers to make "reasonable accommodation" to allow you to function properly in your job.[4]

- The Family Medical Leave Act (FMLA) entitles employees to up to twelve weeks unpaid leave, which can be taken in small increments. This is useful if you have to go to medical appointments.

If you think that your co-workers are treating you unfairly, talk to the boss. If the boss is treating you unfairly, contact a medical social worker, or a local office of a cancer organization for information about your rights and other support.

When you are off work, keep in touch with colleagues to inform them of your progress. Side effects of treatment may require you to be at home but you may still be able to do part-time work.

ABOUT FUTURE CHOICES AND THE LAW

Legal papers, known as **advanced directives**, make your wishes clear about end-of-life health care and about what you wish to pass onto your loved ones. They ensure your wishes are as binding as possible concerning your future.

Legal documents include:

Health care proxy—delegating authority to another person to make health care decisions on your behalf, if you become mentally or physically incapacitated.

Living will—expressing your wishes, to guide your healthcare proxy, as to what your medical treatment should be. For example, you might wish to receive all possible medical interventions or you might refuse treatment that will artificially prolong your life. As previously stated, it's your right to decide to request or refuse treatment as a mentally competent adult.

Granting power of attorney—for non-health issues such as financial and other personal matters.

Writing a will or creating a trust—transferring your assets in accordance with your desires as opposed to your assets being transferred pursuant to state law.

Consult an attorney about the various forms these take and how they apply to you.[5]

Preparing advanced directives does not mean you are about to die

It is important to feel positive about your treatment, but ultimately life does end. Ten out of ten people die. Now is just a good time to stop postponing if, for example, you don't yet have a living will, healthcare proxy or will. Life will be much easier for your beloved family and friends later if they know your wishes about end of life care, the kind of memorial you would like and other preferences.

Joyce *My father who, as a minister, had seen many families troubled by the sudden death and lack of foresight of a spouse, vowed he would have everything in order when he died. He was true to his word. We knew about his will, where to find his bankbooks and other papers, and the funeral arrangements that he had already made and paid for. He even had chosen the hymns to be sung at his funeral service—right down to "omit verse 4!" His pre-planning was a great relief to all of us.*

Whether your first treatment is entirely successful, whether you experience a recurrence, or are constantly having tests to monitor the possibility—*in all cases, preparing advance directives is highly recommended*.

How to put advanced directives in place

Some legal documents may need a lawyer to ensure they are in accordance with state laws and court precedents. It is wise to check as such documents are based on state law, not federal law.

- It is possible to download forms that will be honored as legal if properly signed.
- I highly recommend that you check out both the American Bar Association online toolkit and also especially *Five Wishes* from Aging with Wisdom [6]
- Give a copy of your living will to all significant family members, your doctors, your healthcare proxy and your lawyer. Make sure *everyone* knows about your decision to accept or decline treatment that will artificially prolong your life. It simply isn't enough to sign a living will and have it filed away.

- List where you keep these important documents on the last page of your *Yellow Pages*.

Other advanced directives (not binding)

You may wish to use your recuperation to create several non-legal projects. These might include what is now known as an "ethical will" and/or letters to be given at a later date to loved ones: [7]

Ethical will: You can bequeath your valuable heartfelt thoughts to other people, not just your money and your worldly goods. You can express your love and share your beliefs or you can pass on the legacy of what you have learned throughout your life: in other words—all the things that money can't buy. The current term for this "ethical will" may be new, but it's not a new idea. It has been around since Biblical times when, before death, a father passed on not only his wisdom and blessing to his son, but practical burial instructions and even prophecies about the future.

Other projects: You might enjoy the process of involving family members in family heritage projects such as a photo album to be passed on to a younger generation, or share stories from your past on CD, video or DVD. This too can contribute to your healing.

Anne *When my mother was ill, my father, my brother and I gathered old family pictures together and sat round the fire, sharing memories from long ago. It was most heartwarming to hear some of her stories for the first time. We encouraged her to write her early memories for her grandchildren. After she died, I found a scant four pages. Tucked between her sewing and knitting patterns, they clearly expressed her spirit and reflected her values. We all wished there had been more—and that we had taken more time for such projects years ago.*

- Walk around your home earmarking objects to be gifted to loved ones. Make notes or write a letter about the origin and meaning of each item and perhaps why you would like a particular family member or friend to receive it. You will then be ready to offer these gifts anytime you wish, perhaps in celebration of your return to health.

- Whenever you wish an item to go to a specific individual, make that known to your legal representative and note it in your will or trust—even if it is as simple as "All items with blue 'stickies' go to A___, and all items with red 'stickies' go to B____."

Section 5: Information About Cancer—For Those Who Want to Be Up-to-date

There is a lot of information out there that you may find relevant and interesting. However, this abundance comes in all shapes and sizes. It can be overpowering and possibly incorrect. If you are a person who is reassured by having a lot of information, you will be comfortable gathering it. **If you are easily overwhelmed by lots of facts and figures, delegate this task to someone else.**

How to organize your information about cancer

Start to collect resources *at your own pace.*

Your resources might include:
- Cancer articles
- Book and book references
- Research reports
- Internet search engines, sources and information
- Health organizations
- Community organizations
- Sources of less expensive vitamins, organic produce, drugs
- Humor: movies, cartoons etc. to make you laugh
- Newsletters and blogs
- Personal anecdotes

Initially, you'll be able to put the material at the back of your binder. Quite soon, though, you may find it necessary to sort it according to topic and place it in folders, file boxes or filing cabinet drawers **marking tabs accordingly.**
- If you are interested in, or are combining, both mainstream medicine and complementary care, divide your informa-

tion into two parts: one for mainstream and another for complementary.

- If you are seeing an integrative doctor, keep both parts together.

Refer to *Appendix 2: Directory of Resources* which contain a useful, but limited, number of suggestions about cancer in general, and about creating wellness. It is organized in the following six sections:

1. Organizations & Websites
2. Newsletters, Magazines & Blogs
3. Books
4. Audios & Videos
5. Consulting, Treatment Information & Referral Services
6. Miscellaneous Resources

About Using the Internet

The Internet gives you access to resources and also to companionship through online chat-rooms—for example, of specific cancer organizations.

If you use an Internet search engine, such as Google, you will be amazed and probably dazed at the vast number of possible answers to your query. Searching the internet is a good way to track down a resource if, for example, you only have the name of an author or a title. Your local librarian or bookseller can also be helpful.

If you want to track down books about specific cancers, www.Amazon.com is helpful. By far the greatest number of books targeting specific cancers have been written about breast cancer, with far fewer about prostate and lung cancer, and fewer still about lymphoma, ovarian and pancreatic cancer, brain tumors, and non-Hodgkins lymphoma.

- **Be cautious.** Websites in particular frequently change their information. What you see one day may not be what is on the screen a week later. Information, called "research," may turn out to be the opinion of one person only, or industry-biased. Or it may be dated. New research is constantly re-shaping treatments that have been state-of-the-art, and sometimes it takes a while for practitioners to catch up with research. So check to see who has sponsored a site and the date of the information given. Is it old or is it so new that it has not yet been verified?

- Refer to the *MEDLINEplus* site in *Appendix 2: Cancer Resources* for helpful guidelines for evaluating websites and healthy web surfing.

You have it in your power, with help from friends, survivors, cancer care professionals, and librarians, to find and analyze information so that you can select whatever is appropriate to you.

Section 6: Personal Contacts, Support and Writing

In this section of your binder, you may want to include notes concerning conversations with family, friends, and support group members, as well as your written responses to explorations in Chapters 2, 7, 8, 9 and 10.

How to organize your personal papers

- Decide how you would like to divide this material. Prepare small-tabbed sub-dividers and arrange it accordingly.
- To refresh your memory about personal writing, refer to Chapter 7, Section 7: *Write From the Heart— Create Your Own Journal*. If your writing is very personal, you may want to keep it in a separate book in a safe place where others will not have access to it.

Since a picture can say more that a thousand words, your personal record may be visual. Tona kept a journal of drawings and cartoons of her medical visits, while Phyllis took photographs. She included snapshots of herself before, during, and after chemotherapy as well as photos of her medical team culled from hospital ads. That way she could see her progress and feel the support of her team.

Section 7: My *Yellow Pages*

Follow the guidelines in Chapter 5 and in Appendix I.

WHEN YOUR PAPERS BULGE AT THE SEAMS— REORGANIZE!

I got impatient when my giant binder became over-stuffed and unwieldy, within months rather than years! It was difficult to take pages in and out. I found a number of separate medium sized binders were preferable in addition to the colorful array of file boxes for all the cancer resources I collected. Some people, like Phyllis, on the other hand, favor one enormous binder where they know they have everything together. Others prefer folders or files in a cabinet.

Here's One Way to Evolve Your System:

Before unruly papers within your original binder begin to overflow, simply transfer the bulging sections into separate binder-books as needed, for example:

Book 1: Western medicine appointments and reports

Book 2: Complementary and alternative medicine visits and reports

Book 3: Financial and legal records

Book 4: Personal papers and writing

Or Get one huge binder!

Time to Throw Out?

As you re-organize, look with fresh eyes at what you have accumulated.

- Is it time to trim down?
- Are you willing to get rid of excess information you no longer need?
- Perhaps someone else could use it?
- Think of getting rid of paperwork clutter as a healthy enterprise. It can help you lighten up!
- Check with an accountant, tax person or lawyer about the length of time required by law to keep financial or legal records, before you throw them out.

🪷 Please note: You can make your task easier with a custom designed binder for *My Hope & Focus Cancer Organizer*. Now available from RootsnWings.com/cancer-organizer

Reach In—
Create Your Own
Wellness Program

～～～ REACH IN

7

Seven Ways to
Enhance Your Healing

Quiet Space and Quality Time

YOU ARE UNIQUE AND YOUR WAY OF WEAVING A PATH through your cancer experience may be different from anyone else's. No matter how much support you get from others, it is important to *care for yourself* in nourishing ways as you make decisions and undergo treatment. You really are your own best friend. Don't allow the disease to become your identity.

Among the many challenges facing you is the need to "be" not only to "do." By putting aside periods each day to slow down, you will be able to give yourself the opportunity to become more fully aware of what you are actually experiencing from moment to moment. Quality time for "being" can open the door to your heart and your own ways of knowing.

It may be difficult to carve out time for yourself when you are caught up in many activities and worries following the diagnosis, but it is a lifeline to health. As you listen to your heart, your inner voice and your gut reactions, you'll know more clearly how you feel, who really supports you, and what course of treatment is in line with your needs and perspectives. By exploring some of the ways to enhance healing, you'll be able to bring balance to your life, replenish your energy, and renew your spirit.

Each one of the health-supporting practices following this introduction has been of benefit to me. Create your own wellness prescription by experimenting with the suggestions that appeal to you. Leave the rest. "Bypass that which you do not love" is advice from ancient wisdom to avoid diversions that dissipate healing powers. Not all the ways to enhance healing will work equally well for everyone.

It's ideal if you can find an environment with as few distractions as possible for times of reflection and exploration. An atmosphere of peace and quiet is most conducive.

- While at home, turn off the telephone, cell phone, TV and computer.

- When you wish to have uninterrupted time for something you love to do, hang a sign on the door handle, saying, "Please don't disturb".

"Bypass that which you do not love" is advice from ancient wisdom to avoid diversions that dissipate healing powers.

- Look for a place or several different places in the neighborhood to sit or walk without intrusion.

- Think about the rhythm of your week. Are there natural breaks in your schedule when you can put aside routine tasks—daily? Weekly? There's great wisdom in the ancient practice of taking a complete day of rest every seventh day.

- Live life as fully as possible so that you don't become solely identified with the disease. Become involved with a group having little or nothing to do with your healing, but which interests you. For example, if you love to connect with children but do not, offer to volunteer at a children's reading program at your local library. Sometimes it helps to change perspectives and consciousness by changing the environment.

There may be days when you are physically depleted from appointments or treatments and when your body needs to rest in order to amplify its own healing energies. It is always good to respect that need. **Rest and relaxation support healing at every level**—body, mind, emotions and spirit.

1. Relax ... More Often

Here's what relaxation can do:

- Relaxation is good for the body. It reduces muscle tensions and cramps, lowers the heart rate and blood pressure and helps to recharge and balance physical energy.
- Relaxation is good for the mind. It enhances the functioning of the brain and nervous system and improves the quality of thoughts and images.
- Relaxation is good for emotions. As you become more centered, it is easier to let go of worry, and release extreme, disturbing or painful feelings.
- Relaxation is good for the spirit. It can open your inner vision and inspire you to appreciate the wonders of life.

First of all, get enough sleep and plenty of fresh air. We often take breathing for granted yet, for centuries, regulating the breath has been one of the simplest and most frequently-used methods of becoming relaxed in almost all cultures. Learning to let go of tensions is an important key to health. Studies show that when relaxation increases, stress lessens. As you relax you return to a more natural state in which you can become more present in the moment, rather than uptight and goal-oriented, fearing the future or crying over the spilt milk of the past.

In 1975, Herbert Benson, MD, outlined both the physiology that led to illnesses caused by stress and what to do about it. "Each of us," he said, "possesses a natural and innate protective mechanism against overstress." This he termed the "relaxation response."[1] You can call on it to deal with difficult situations and enhance your well-being. There are four essential elements—a quiet environment, a mental device such as a word or a phrase, which should be repeated over and over again, or an object to gaze on, a receptive attitude and a comfortable position.

Mary *I learned to relax so I could listen to my body. If I was tense, I didn't know what treatments were good for me. If I relaxed, nine times out of ten I could tell what was right for me. Don't let other people tell you what to do or not to do. Relax first and then listen to your own body. Really trust your body.*

Try one or several of these ways of relaxing

REST

Put your feet up or take a nap. Let out some sighs and some big yawns. If your energy dips in the afternoon, lie flat on your back after lunch. Simply rest. This is good for the internal organs. For help in falling asleep, choose a CD or downloadable MP3 that encourages deep sleep for half an hour such as the Catnapper in the *Timeout Hemi-Sync* series.[2]

RELEASE PHYSICAL TENSION

- Tighten parts of the body and then release quickly—the arms, shoulders, legs, etc., then the whole body.
- Make a really tight clenched fist, quickly release the tension by stretching your fingers out. Repeat several times.
- Shake your arms and legs in turn to release any tension held in the joints.
- Gently circle ankles, wrists, elbows, shoulders and head.
- In the shower gently massage your neck and shoulders and take some extra time to massage your head.

BREATHE

- Stop what you are doing, sit or lie quietly and notice how you are breathing.
  - ~ Focus only on the rhythm of the breath as you breathe in and out. Put your hand on your chest or abdomen and feel it rise and fall.
  - ~ Then, deepen and slow down your breath while you sink into a rhythm of greater calm.
  - ~ Or create a circle of acceptance, comfort and relaxation by putting one hand on your heart and one hand on your abdomen as you breathe gently.
  - ~ Or as you breathe in silently say, "I calm my body," and as you breath out silently say, "I smile," as Thich Nhat Hanh suggests; or shorten it to: breathing in—"calm," breathing out—"smile." You can do it anywhere.

ACTIVATE YOUR RELAXATION RESPONSE

- Sit passively in a comfortable quiet environment, focus on repeating a word such as "peace" over and over again, or look at a still object.

2. Use Guided Imagery to Your Advantage

GUIDED IMAGERY IS A VERY EMPOWERING TOOL

Listening to guided imagery or creative visualization audios (MP3s, CDs or DVDs) can increase health, lead to experiencing a specific feeling such as tranquility, deepen relaxation and bring balance to the body, mind, emotions and spirit. Both the music and tone of voice are designed to relax you and then engage the power of your imagination. Through the use of selected images, you can focus very specifically and purposefully towards a chosen goal, since imagery precedes action.

Many audios are specifically designed for healing.[3] Some use imagery with the intention of amplifying healing in conjunction with surgery,[4] chemotherapy or radiation; others address stress reduction and general wellness. Imagery can also reduce high blood pressure and boost the immune system. In their pioneering work with imagery, Drs. Carl and Stephanie Simonton encouraged their patients to have a clear understanding of the physical processes in their illnesses as well as a clear sense of the ideal outcome of their treatments.[5] Research shows that medically correct imagery, for example imagining the body's T-cells and killer cells removing the cancer, is most helpful. Some people do better with symbols, visualizing the healing forces as small cranes removing small boxes of poison (the cancer cells).

Research shows that medically correct imagery, for example imagining the body's T-cells and killer cells removing the cancer, is most helpful.

CHOOSE IMAGERY THAT WORKS FOR YOU

Garrett was nine when he was diagnosed with an inoperable brain tumor. He first received radiation until further treatments were no longer safe. Although his prognosis was terminal, he made a decision to do everything he could to live, and with the help of his biofeedback therapist, he embarked on an all out war against his tumor.[6] Following in the Simontons' footsteps, his therapist introduced visualization and relaxation techniques. In Garrett's opinion, the imagery she suggested was too boring for kids. Since he loved *Star Trek*, he proceeded to create, with her help, an action-packed space war against his tumor. They made an audio that he felt could be of use to others too. Garrett could mentally "see" his tumor as he used the visualizations. He persevered, for at least a year, in his determination to get well and then, one day, he could no longer see his tumor. A CAT scan later confirmed that the tumor was gone.[7] This courageous boy went on to set up a local telephone hotline for children with cancer.[8]

Marion Woodman, PhD, used imagery differently when cancer entered her life in her mature years. She wrote in her journal, "I put my own hot hands on my belly and bring in light and heat. I'm no good at *fighting* cancer cells. I can't use a gun or wild dogs or spitfires. Those images do not work for me, but I can suffuse darkness with light, and I do, three or four times a day, and often in the night."[9]

Puja I tend to play my favorite guided imagery audios over and over again.[10] Some have both imagery and affirmations. When I was diagnosed, I used an image-specific audio for cancer and guided imagery created especially for me. At the time of my lumpectomy I listened to a tape for surgery. Later I experimented with something new—listening to a series of meditation CDs using technology that utilizes the latest research in sound waves and brain waves to create a shift in consciousness.[11] While listening to these CDs, I could at the same time use breathing techniques or pray.

Visualization works best when you are able to relax, at a time and in a place without the pressure of external demands. My favorite time is after lunch but you will discover your own best times. It's better to ease gently into imagery rather than grab or force it. If you surrender to the guidance of the words and background music, you will be able to enter a deeply relaxed, diffuse state, where the psyche will provide your own images of what is being suggested. You will be encouraged to use many senses: seeing, hearing, smelling, touching, even tasting. Research studies show that visualization with this whole-body sense of what you are imagining can have a very powerful effect. Your body actually has the capacity to become more peaceful and refreshed, as if it were actually in the situation you are imagining.

Visualization works best when you are able to relax, at a time and in a place without the pressure of external demands.

The imagery in the first exploration to follow is designed to help you become more grounded. Allow a picture of a tree or plant to emerge that is appealing. In the second, when asked to choose a place that feels very safe and nourishing, trust your intuition to take you there. It could be familiar or unfamiliar, perhaps a place outdoors in nature that you have visited, or a special building that you love. Or it may be an imaginary place that feels very special and comforting.

For some people imagery is easy. If you are among those who can't quite seem to focus or quiet the mind enough to become aware of imagery, don't worry. It is a skill that develops over time with practice.

Before You Begin any Guided Imagery

- Turn off the ringer on the phone and ask not to be disturbed.
- Sit comfortably in a chair or lie on your bed.
- Shut your eyes and let go into a few deep, full, cleansing breaths. Or, do some quiet centering.

Imagery to Become More Grounded

- Put your hand on your heart or belly, a place where you can feel the breath coming in and out.
- From there, imagine, visualize or sense that you are getting in touch with a pathway for energy to flow down your body and legs, connecting through your feet with the earth.
- Imagine that the pathway extends from your feet deep into the earth. Feel and smell the earth beneath your feet. Sense that your connection is helping to anchor you firmly in the earth and is spreading out and opening to receive the earth's rich nourishment.
- When you feel your "roots" have gone deep enough, invite earth's comfort and calm to come up through this pathway to strengthen you. Imagine it is filling your feet first, then your legs and then your whole body. Feel yourself becoming more centered and well-grounded as you willingly allow yourself to be replenished.
- If you wish, invite a picture of yourself as a healthy strong tree or beautiful plant.
- As you breathe slowly in and out, let yourself fully absorb the qualities of this tree or plant—its strength, beauty, deli-

Try these guided imagery explorations

cacy or vibrancy. Note how you feel, where you are and what season it is.

Give yourself a Relaxing Mini-vacation in a Safe Space

Settle quietly, with your eyes shut.

- Set the condition that you will only go to a place or situation that feels very nourishing and safe for you where you can let go of burdens you are carrying. Go wherever your inner self wants to take you, trusting that it will be healing.

  For example, you could lean against a tree that supports you, lie on a rock that absorbs your negativity, or climb to the top of a mountain where you can get a higher perspective.

- Through your gentle breathing, continue to release any tensions you no longer want and no longer need. Feel them melting away. You may even see them going out through the surface of your skin and into the air around you, not to return. Open up to the sounds, smells and the feeling of the place or situation you have chosen.

  For those who love being beside the ocean:

- Call to mind your favorite beach, or create an imaginary beach in your mind. See yourself comfortably sitting in your beach chair, lying on your blanket on the sand or floating on the calm water. As you relax more and more, feel the sun and warm wind on your skin; hear the rhythmic sound of the waves as they reach the shore, and even taste the sea salt on your lips. Look at the soft contours of the horizon and let yourself be cradled in its peaceful expanse, or enjoy the play of light on the water or on your skin. You have nothing else to do and nowhere else to be for these moments. Let yourself fully absorb the energy of land, water and sky as you breathe slowly in and out.

Other Choices

- Find one or two audios you like and use them regularly so your healing intention becomes stronger over time.
- Ask a hypnotherapist to custom design a personal audio with specific imagery and affirmations for you.

- Invite your mind to come up with imagery, symbolic or physiological, to address the issue you have chosen to work on.

3. Be Open to Creativity

Whether you appreciate the beauty others have created or create beauty as an expressive outlet for your own imagination, it is now known that such activities have healing, nurturing power. Through creativity you can become more aware and connected to the beauty or wonder of the world—and of yourself. The form may vary greatly—from drawing, woodwork and gardening to mask making, stamp collecting and dancing. If there is something you've always wanted to do, and your treatment doesn't yet allow it, dream about it. Then, as you become stronger, take preliminary steps so that you will be ready to put the dream fully into action when you feel sufficiently fit. Below I've chosen music, art and color as examples.

MUSIC

It goes without saying that music affects people at a very deep level. This is true both for the outdoor music of nature, such as birdsong or crickets, and for music played on instruments or from the human voice. Music's language is universal. It can shift your mood in an instant, inspiring you to march, sing or dance to the rhythm of a beat. It can conjure up happy memories and move you to tears.

Music's great potential for healing human conditions has been known and used since ancient times. Studies verify that the frequency and vibration of music can produce very specific positive results. For example, it has been shown that the waltz, coming from the ancient Sufi tradition, opens the heart. Listening to Mozart is of great benefit to those who suffer from depression. Baroque music stimulates the capacity to concentrate and retain knowledge from reading. Studies even reveal that some classical music increases the growth of plants and the milk-yield of cows. So it is well worth listening to music you love while on your healing journey.[12]

You may want to make your own music. Perhaps you enjoyed playing the piano or another instrument a long time ago. It may be time to return to such old loves if you left them behind in the course of your life. If you love to sing, sing in your car or with friends, join a choir or simply sing in the shower.

ART AND COLOR

When I was considering what my wellness program might include, I remembered a saying I was told a long time ago—"A drawing a day keeps the doctor away." I found it empowering to express and release my feelings non-verbally and spontaneously with colored crayons on paper. To shut off my inner critic, I sometimes closed my eyes as I drew, or I drew with my non-dominant hand. It didn't matter to me that some of my drawings were quite raw. That was not the point. No one else was going to see them.

Your creativity need not be beautiful, artistic or perfect. Many people enjoy the sensation of molding clay, building sand sculptures, or mixing colors together with wet paint, preferring the process rather than the finished product. Use colors that express your mood in your artwork, and pay attention to the color of clothes you like to wear. Color itself has great healing potential to bring balance.[13] Every color has a vibration so allow your attraction to colors to change—as you do.

- Remember a hobby or some kind of creativity you enjoyed as a child. Let yourself play with that again in the spirit of a child.

- Find a creativity group you'd enjoy in which you will learn something new.

- Play waltz music and allow it to open your heart. If you can, dance.

- Play baroque music while you are preparing for a medical visit to help you focus.

- As you listen to classical music allow it to flow right into the area of your body that is in need of healing.

- Sing along with the music you love.

- Every day choose some colored crayons and let your hands freely express your mood.

- Enjoy your favorite art-form.

Try one of these ways of enjoying creativity

4. Keep Your Energy Flowing—With Movement, Diet and Bodywork

WHY IS IT SO IMPORTANT TO KEEP YOUR ENERGY MOVING?

Like a stream that no longer moves, energy can become stagnant and polluted. This is not good for health. In 1995, with over twenty years of research at the University of California at Los Angeles under her belt, Dr. Valerie Hunt, PhD, first recorded energy changes in action in healing sessions, such as Rolfing, with sophisticated tracking technology. She wrote, "As a result of my work I can no longer consider the body as organic systems or tissues. The healthy body is a flowing interactive electro-dynamic energy field. Motion is more natural to life than non-motion—things that keep flowing are inherently good. What interferes with flow will have detrimental effects."[14]

Many complementary practitioners believe that it is a healthy practice to invite a strong current of "life-force" or "chi" to move through the body since any depleted, stuck or blocked energy can manifest in symptoms of illness such as depression, back pain, cancer or anxiety.

Unfortunately we now live in an inherently unhealthy environment. The air is not pure, the water is not clean, and our cleaning products, cosmetics and food are largely contaminated with pesticides, herbicides, fungicides, preservatives and toxic chemicals. These contaminants stress the body's ability to function at optimum capacity. Day in and day out our systems have to work harder to deal with carcinogens and the many other tainted substances taken into our bodies through the nose, mouth and skin. None of us can escape this planetary health crisis, but we can make healthy choices wherever possible.

Exercise, nutrition and bodywork are extremely important complementary adjuncts to any treatment plan you choose.

- Exercise, nutrition and bodywork are extremely important complementary adjuncts to any treatment plan you choose.
- Exercise oxygenates the body, stimulates the lymphatic system and increases circulation. Lack of activity has been identified as a risk factor for (breast) cancer recurrence and mortality.
- Natural supplements can be helpful to build bodily strength.
- To minimize the pesticides, hormones and antibiotics entering your system, buy organic fruit, veggies, eggs, dairy products and meats. Cut out non-organic food, wherever possible, but do add prebiotics and probiotics to support the healthy bacteria in your gut. New research indicates supporting your microbiome is fundamental to health. Don't stop there. Anything you put on your hair, nails, scalp or skin is absorbed into your body like a food, so check cosmetic labels for "parabens" and "phthalates."[15] Check household cleaning products for chlorine bleach, and become aware of other toxic chemicals and pesticides used in the environment. Avoid using plastics or plastic wrap around food when you cook them in the microwave. Dioxin carcinogens from the plastic can leach into your food, especially into fats, and from there they go directly into your body. Instead, use tempered glass, Corning Ware or ceramic containers.

"A good massage will lower blood pressure, reduce heart rate and have all kinds of beneficial physiologic effects. It also relaxes muscles and, in a circular fashion, relieves distress."[16] While it is difficult to find even one solid randomized, double-blind study that stands up to rigorous scientific research, there are lots of less rigorous studies, patient surveys and anecdotal information that point to the benefits of massage for cancer patients, especially with regard to the symptoms of treatment.[17]

Other forms of hands-on energy work can help you to relax more deeply into your body, mind and spirit. All contribute greatly to stress reduction. This is very important, since the more stressed you are, the higher the level of the stress hormone, cortisol, is likely to be. A high level can wreak havoc with the immune system response, reducing wanted natural killer cell activation, thus weakening the body's ability to clean out mutant cancerous cells.

Remember, activities that keep your energy flowing are good for you.

Puja   *I have three favorite ways of keeping my energy flowing through my body: The first is exercise. I love to walk, play tennis, and swim in summer. I use a form of weights called Smartbells[18] and cross-country ski in winter. The second is being careful with my diet. I eat healthy foods and constantly have to remind myself to drink plenty of water. (Some doctors believe you need 20% more nutrients after a cancer diagnosis to build strength and repair tissue.) After my diagnosis, I became far more conscious of the need to eat organic products and to limit favorite sugar treats like sweet desserts and cookies as much as possible. Thirdly, I love to be at the receiving end of a massage or energy balancing healing when I do nothing but lie there. Likewise I can lie on my back on the floor when I use my exerciser 2000, a machine that vibrates my legs and increases my oxygenation. I found that using a sauna regularly also helps detoxify my body while I am relaxing. Afterwards I feel squeaky-clean. It is easier to follow through on activities that are enjoyable as well as healthy.*

Try one of these ways of keeping your energy flowing

WITH EXERCISE

- Do simple stretches when you get up in the morning.
- Walk every day. Include some brisk walking.
- Join a yoga or tai chi class. Or choose some form of aerobic exercise.
- Start slowly if you have not been accustomed to strenuous exercise.

WITH GOOD NUTRITION

- Go organic.
- Drink 6-8 + glasses of water per day.
- Cut back on sugar and processed foods or better still cut them out.
- Read labels of food, cosmetic and household products for synthetic and artificial ingredients, and genetically modified foods. Buy accordingly.
- Become aware of the vitamin and mineral supplements your body needs. Natural vitamins are more easily absorbed and can support health whereas synthetic vitamins may actually stress the body. To be safe, consult a health professional.

WITH BODYWORK

- Make an appointment for your favorite treatment.
    - ~ If you enjoy your feet being touched, request a reflexology session.
    - ~ If you like a light touch, request a cranial-sacral session.
    - ~ If you want to feel deeply relaxed request a polarity session, and so on.
- Try a treatment you have never had.
- Ask for lymphatic drainage within a massage.

5. Connect With Nature

NATURE'S GIFTS

Nature keeps us in touch with the miracle of the seasons and cycles of life—natural rhythms that remind us of our place in the larger scheme of things. What a blessing! Einstein reminds us, "There are two ways to live your life—one as though nothing is a miracle. The other is as though everything is a miracle."[19] Connecting with nature can help us participate in miracles.

Sunsets don't cost anything. Nor do sunrises, starry nights, fireflies, the first snowdrop, the exuberance of fall colors, or the smell of honeysuckle. Mother Earth showers her abundance on us, whether we pay attention or not. It's easy to take her gifts for granted. Far too often we've been taught to treat the earth as an object to be controlled and used with no contemplation of her mysteries. We need not do so. When we get on board with the current scientific understanding that everything that exists is energy pulsating, we can appreciate that the earth is not just physical matter to be manipulated.[20] Nature's vibrant energy can contribute powerfully to our healing not only emotionally and spiritually, but also physically.

Enjoying nature can be comforting even if you are not able to go outdoors. When I have to remain indoors, I love to watch the sun going down, looking out from a comfortable chair. It's a magical time. I appreciate my houseplants, photos of beautiful places and guided imagery audios set in nature.

When I have been speeding through life and have become fragmented in one of my tizzies, I go for a walk, or sit or lie in the grass under a tree. I know it's time for nature's healing presence to slow me down and connect me again to my essential being.

OUTDOORS

Try one of these ways of enjoying nature

- Find a peaceful spot and just sit there. Let illness bring the opportunity to connect to simple pleasures such as taking deep breaths of fresh air.
- Walk as much or as little as you are able—anywhere, in your yard, your neighborhood, a public park or preserve.
- Sit with your back against a tree. Feel and absorb its support.
- Listen to the water of a flowing stream. As you relax into listening, become aware of both its many different sounds and the harmony of the whole.

- In summer, lie on the grass and place whatever part of your body is hurting or tight against the ground. Pay attention to the contact with the earth as you gently breath and allow the earth's energy to be absorbed into your body.
- Ask someone to take you for a drive if you are not able to do so yourself.
- Feel the wind on your hair.
- Look up at a starry night sky.
- Linger as you look into a favorite flower.

INDOORS

To bring the peace of nature into your life indoors, you might:
- Listen to a CD or MP3 of ocean sounds or birdcalls. Let yourself drift off on a journey prompted by the nature sounds.
- Appreciate a beautiful houseplant, or a vase of freshly cut flowers. Smell, touch, linger…
- Look at a painting or a photograph of beautiful natural surroundings.
- Look out of the window from your bed or a comfortable chair. If there are no trees, look at the sky and the play of light at different times of day and in different weather, perhaps sunrise and sunset.

6. Lighten Your Mood—Do Things That Bring You Pleasure

One of the first questions I asked my doctors after my surgery was 'When can I play tennis again?'

If you take care of yourself in ways that give you joy, you'll be stronger for all the hard work surrounding your cancer treatment. Weaving pleasure into your life, be it simple appreciation of nature or a favorite activity, is life-affirming. Garden, swim, play chess, watch a ball game, embroider, create a picture, sing or choose any other activity that sparks your passion. This will lighten your mood. Let your love of an activity serve as an incentive to get you back to health.

Welcoming pleasure can be an important step for those who are habitual self-deniers. If this is the case with you, it may be good to give yourself permission to learn something new that has intrigued you for years. If you have been stingy with yourself, spend money on a vacation or on something beautiful that brings you joy.

Like nature's gifts that cost nothing, a smile, a hug, a word of thanks and "random acts of kindness" are free and easy to do. They can lighten the spirit of both the giver and the receiver.

Laughter too has long been recognized to be enormously healing, so keep your sense of humor alive by renting or going to movies that make you laugh, as Norman Cousins did.[21] A good belly laugh can boost the immune system: it increases the number of natural killer cells that can attack certain kinds of cancer and decreases stress hormones. It is also good for the cardiovascular system: It can increase heart rate and blood pressure similar to aerobic exercise.

If You Can't Do it Now, Envision it

Even if you can't do some of the things you love now, hold onto a positive vision of how you'd like to live your life after the difficult times of your treatment. This will actually help you. It will strengthen your courage and influence your healing *now*. In a remarkable book, author Victor Frankl documents how even in the horrendous conditions of the Nazi concentration camps those prisoners who had something to look forward to, which gave their life meaning, such as writing a manuscript or reuniting with a loved one, were much more likely to survive.[22]

Welcome the dreams of how you would like to be or what you would like to do once you have recuperated...

Welcome the dreams of how you would like to be or what you would like to do once you have recuperated, and explore how you might manifest them. But, also be sure you're not underestimating what you are capable of now. Give it a try. Stretch yourself. You might be surprised at how healing this can be, if done with sensitivity. Lawrence LeShan found that when people were in extreme cancer crisis, if he pushed them as hard as possible for their lives—within the parameters of their preferences, rather than backing off to accommodate the cancer crisis—they would often begin to get better. [23]

Try some of these ways of giving yourself pleasure

- Pamper yourself—treat yourself to a manicure, a pedicure, or something else that will make you feel good.
- Rent, or go to a movie that will make you laugh.
- Check out www.colorsinmotion.com/touchstone.html
- Take a friend out for a special dinner.
- Do something out of character that you suspect might be a lot of fun.
- Slow down and enjoy whatever is around you. Pet your cat.
- Ask for a hug; give a hug.
- Connect with a child.
- Dream.

7. Write From Your Heart–Create Your Own Journal

THE BENEFITS OF PERSONAL WRITING

Remember how wonderful it feels to be warmly welcomed with open arms by another! I love that feeling. In a split second, the power of the affectionate gesture comes flooding into you straight from the heart of your loving friend. When you take time to write to yourself with honesty and innocence from your heart, you are extending a similar gesture of openness and love towards yourself.

The act of writing freely about what is happening in your life can be profoundly significant. Writing gives you time for reflection, and thinking about what you have written may slow you down a bit and give you fresh insights. You may well discover that you are expressing much more than you expected, surprising even yourself.

COMMUNICATING TO AND FROM YOUR INNER SELF

First, choose a suitable book for your personal writing. Some people like to use a beautiful blank notebook, or one with a saying for the day or a little drawing on each page, so that it is clearly different from other kinds of writing or record-keeping. Others prefer to write on loose-leaf paper, which they can add, sheet by sheet, to a journal binder later, so that they don't have to carry it all around.

Use the suggestions on the following page, like warming-up exercises at the gym, to get you started and loosen up your writing ability. As you respond to the suggestions, you'll be developing the knack of communicating—to and from your inner self. Let your thoughts and feelings flow onto the page; then edit it later if you wish. Personal writing reflects *your* inner experience—however you wish to express it.

What and how you write may depend on many things— on your mood, what you are currently experiencing in your treatment, or how much energy you have. At times you may find yourself completing a brief sentence or even drawing a blank. At other times you may write quickly and furiously because you can hardly keep up with all the thoughts and feelings that are tumbling out of you. Or you may reach for your crayons or colored markers because you want to express a mood without words.

I found that writing from my heart brought comfort, companionship, inspiration and challenge on my pilgrimage to health.

Each in your own way, you may embark on a rich inward journey where the person you get to know is *you.* Note the date and anything else that affects the writing process so that over time you get an overview of how simultaneously you are building a foundation to support you from beneath and gaining a new perspective from above.

THE IMPORTANCE OF PRIVACY

Whether your personal writing is in a three-ring binder or a beautifully bound book, be sure to keep it in a safe space, separate from your medical records. Make a pact with yourself that you are writing for yourself alone so you can really be honest—especially if you might be tempted to alter what you write in case others might read it. If you do decide to share any of your writing, you can at that point choose to edit it as needed.

Try these ways of writing freely from your heart

AT ANY TIME OF DAY OR NIGHT

- Sit quietly with a blank sheet of paper, a beautiful notebook or your journal in front of you. Note the date.
- Breathe gently and when you are ready, allow your thoughts and feelings to flow from your heart through your hands on to the paper in *this* moment.
- Express yourself freely in whatever way you wish—write, draw with colored crayons pens or pencils. Add additional pages as needed.

AT THE END OF THE DAY

- Become aware of both what has happened during the day, and your feelings about it. Perhaps start by asking questions such as, "How is my treatment plan going? What decisions have I made or do I have to make? What am I thankful for? What am I ready to forgive or ask forgiveness for? And what is left undone?"

IF YOU DO NOT FIND PUTTING PEN TO PAPER EASY

- Review the seven ways to enhance healing in this chapter.
  - ~ Turn to the section which most interests you and follow the train of your thoughts and feelings to wherever they take you.

IF YOU'D LIKE TO TELL STORIES FROM YOUR LIFE

- Choose a theme; for example, write about the things that have given you pleasure, unexpected happenings, or lessons you have learned.
- Consider writing a mini-memoir.

IF YOU'D LIKE TO SHARE YOUR THOUGHTS AND BLESSINGS WITH OTHERS

- Contemplate the special thoughts, blessings and wishes you'd wish to pass on to your loved ones and gently begin to write…

To Sum Up

A personal wellness program is unique to each individual. Here is Esther's:

Esther I made it a practice to read uplifting books and accounts that told stories of successful healing. I used a wonderful tape by Shivani Goodman[24] on a regular basis. I used Kinotakara footpads for detoxification, Master's Miracle Mineral Neutralizer to drink and bathe with to lower acidity and increase PH in my body. I took green drinks and installed a "gizmo" to our water supply to increase alkalinity. I cut out sugar, decaf and processed foods, ate organic and grass-fed meats, milk and vegetables, and drank more water. I made sure to take frequent walks each week regardless of the weather. I took 'The Journey' workshop with Brandon Bays[25] and frequently did her process to release unconscious conflict. I discovered the Yuen Method of Full Spectrum Healing and found this method to be freeing and effective, increasing my sense of over-all well being and health. And I put my spiritual practice back into a primary position."

You may not have heard of all the things that Esther did, but it was right for her. You will find your own way to heal. Trust that. Select your own self-care priorities on the next page.

At a future date, scan through the suggestions in this chapter again and look for those that fit with your situation at that moment. Your program may change over time depending on various circumstances. Bear in mind that it is a choice to contribute as much as you can to your own healing, even if it means letting go of some old habits. A steady ongoing commitment works best. If you can develop the resilience to keep getting through difficulties and even envision yourself thriving, you will be giving your body a powerful message to be well.

**Review
your
self-care
wellness
program**

**I am choosing to enhance my healing by
prioritizing and giving space for the following:**

(Check those that you can commit to at this time)

☐ relaxation

☐ meditation

☐ guided imagery

☐ singing

☐ painting or being creative
   by_____

☐ listening to music

☐ appreciation of beauty

☐ connecting to nature

☐ walking

☐ exercise by _____

☐ wholesome diet

☐ people I love to be with __

☐ things I love to do_____

☐ resurrecting an old hobby

☐ massage and/or body work

☐ eliminating stress

☐ having naps

☐ pampering myself by ___

☐ writing in my journal

☐ dreams—short-term and/
   or long-term goals

☐ laughter

☐ gratitude

☐ movies

☐ gardening

☐ time alone

☐ other ways to love and
   appreciate my life_____

• Make notes about how and when you will follow through
  on these choices.

Heal More Than Your Body—So Your Body Can Heal

1. Body, Mind, Emotions and Spirit —Dynamically Interconnected

THE BODY, MIND, EMOTIONS AND SPIRIT ARE ALL DYNAMI-cally interconnected and involved in the healing process. You can use your mind to recognize and release old self-sabotaging habits and, instead, develop healing attitudes. You can open to deeper feelings, hopes, fears, dreams and intuitions about what is happening through your illness and can nurture your spiritual life to amplify healing. That's what this chapter is all about.

You can use your mind to recognize and release old self-sabotaging habits and, instead, develop healing attitudes.

EVER-MOVING STABILITY

Life is experienced in four ways—through body, mind, emotions and spirit. C. J. Jung referred to these aspects of being as the four "functions"—sensing, thinking, feeling, and intuiting. I find it easy to remember them as the four "h"s—hand, head, heart, and hunch¹—which work together towards health and healing. According to numerology, *four* represents stability and practicality. Nature has four seasons, four phases of the moon and four cardinal directions of the compass reflecting ongoing balance. Each contributes uniquely to the circle of life, in turn predominating, in turn yielding. Seamlessly flowing, they teach us of cycles, cooperation and rhythm. The comfort and strength of *four* appears to be embedded deep within us. Child and adult alike delight in finding that lucky four-leaf clover!

HEALING IS WHOLENESS

The word *heal* and the word *whole* come from the same root—*haleness,* a state of robust good health or completeness to which we can aspire. The phrase *hale and hearty* describes a healthy "whole-hearted" person. I believe we can't get to wholeness through the body alone, through emotions alone, through mind alone, or through spiritual practices alone. Our culture largely teaches us how to separate and compartmentalize, not how to connect and bring balance. In general, we are more comfortable with, and thus over-emphasize, the familiar activities we are proficient at, and which satisfy us. We put all our eggs in that particular basket and neglect the more difficult challenges. This is natural, but it's not healthy when our preference for the familiar leads us to limit or exclude other possibilities. It is wise to pay attention to any part of us that we may have neglected.

Let me illustrate this with regard to health. Have you noticed that people who are good at sports have no trouble working out at the gym whereas those who lead a very sedentary life often resist exercise—even if that is the very thing that is needed to increase their metabolism and health? Or that those who have found safety and praise in being smart, first want to use their heads to think things through very tenaciously, while perhaps ignoring their intuition? Those who rely solely on their feelings to guide them through life most often turn to therapy or groups to bring health even if, by doing so, they might actually be wallowing in their emotions. Likewise people who turn to God and prayer alone to solve all their problems may be totally ignoring their responsibility to evaluate first how their feelings have colored their words or actions, possibly aggravating a problematic situation, and then how they might contribute to a solution.

Cancer patients are continually using the left-brain (rational, logical mind) to sort out information, make decisions and attend to logistical details. It becomes especially important to find time to honor the balancing contribution of the right brain (feeling, integrative mind) and so bring into play intuitive ways of knowing and the capacity to see a bigger picture. Balancing the four functions brings healing and wholeness.

THE BODY'S WISDOM AND HEALING GIFTS

Pain and illness indicate that something is wrong with the physical body. If you didn't know that, you wouldn't take steps to remedy the situation. Dr. Edward Bach[2] used to say, "Illness is already part of the cure." In other words, perhaps we should thank our illness for what it reveals to us. Naturally at the time of my diagnosis, I didn't particularly feel like thanking my cancer. However, knowing that cancerous cells were in my body gave me an opportunity to set up an intention and a plan to deal with it.

A principle called *homeostasis* keeps human beings in a healthy balance by providing early warning signals when we get out of balance. Bodily sensations—an ache, a pain or exhaustion—will reveal what you may have neglected or overused physically. For example, muscles aching from working physically too long and too hard cry out for rest in order to heal and renew. Drinking when thirsty or eating when hungry are other good examples of how everyone instinctively wants to make an adjustment to keep healthy as a result of direct body sensations. In cooperating with these signs, you support the body's natural resilience and preference to be healthy.

Let's go a step further. Since all parts of you are dynamically interconnected, your body may also be telling you that something is out of balance elsewhere—in your thinking, your emotions or your spiritual life. This too is a gift as *any* disparity may eventually contribute to physical illness.

Perhaps, like me, you may have had a headache, not because you bumped into something, but because you had become emotionally tense or mentally exhausted. Or, from time to time, you may have felt sick, not because you have eaten some food that disagreed with you, but because you were in overload and needed time out or because you felt conflicted, angry or resentful. In wanting to throw up, your body was perhaps letting you know you had swallowed (agreed to) something that really didn't sit right and wasn't "good" for you.

BODY AS METAPHOR AND TRUTHFUL BAROMETER

I have learned over the years that if I approach my body as a friend and not an inanimate object, it is very willing to share its wisdom with me.

The connection between emotional stress, physical symptoms and illness has been understood for centuries. Woven into our language are phrases that link a specific bodily pain with a specific feeling. For example "he is a pain in the neck," "she is hard-hearted," and "he has a stiff upper lip" are likely to illustrate aggravation, criticism and stoicism respectively. "She is spineless" or "he has no backbone," may indicate apathy; while "she died of a broken heart" may indicate the connection between heart disease and loss or lack of love.[3] This link between language and the body is quite natural. When the physical body provides clues about emotions, through "heart-felt" feelings and "gut" reactions, pay attention, because this too is part of the miraculous healing process.

I have learned over the years that if I approach my body as a friend and not an inanimate object, it is very willing to share its wisdom with me. Shortly after I was diagnosed, I initiated a silent inner conversation with my body, which I jotted down in my journal as it progressed.

Puja   I asked, "What have I ignored that has contributed to my diagnosis?" I waited quietly for an answer to emerge, not knowing what would come. Much to my surprise, my body replied without a moment's hesitation. It had a lot to say! "Create more healthy boundaries so you can take time for yourself to center and heal. You've been draining yourself for too long. You must strengthen yourself at the core. You are a strong woman, but your bones are the weak link in your genetic chain." (I have osteoporosis.) "You need bone strength, not calcifications in your breast— where it doesn't belong. Let go of anything that bolsters you from the outside in, rather than from the inside out. How about forgiving and releasing all the little hurts, regrets and resentments that still pull you down into the past? They poison your life like the toxicity of accumulated garbage. Perhaps you could do an inventory for forgiveness?"

I'd received my marching orders from within. Much as I might have wanted to ignore some of these painful messages, I could sense the truth they contained. The information I received from my body gave me a chance to reassess and work with my attitudes and emotions to bring healing. Did I want to continue the resentful energy of "It's not fair," a phrase I used a lot as I was growing up? I discovered this theme was still lurking around in my complaints and resentments about my genetic heritage, relationships and the choices I have made. For example, osteoporosis is part of my family's heritage, but why did my twin brother get the hard bones and teeth while I got the soft ones? In intimate relationships with others, I tended to blame the other person for my difficulties, but as a result of body-oriented therapy, such old patterns have eased. I admit however that, under stress, I sometimes revert back to old "whines."

It's a natural phenomenon to regress under great stress. When you become aware of what you are doing, it's better to comfort yourself and pick yourself up again like a child who has fallen, rather than waste energy giving yourself a hard time.

If you reflect on your body's messages in a non-judgmental or meditative way, you may discover insights that will contribute powerfully to healing and you will become healthier in the fullest sense of the word. In addition to using the gift of the body's code to track down and heal imbalances, the rest of the chapter shows you how to use the gifts of your mind, emotions and spirit to bring healing closer.

2. How You Think is How You Heal—How Your Mind Contributes to Healing Your Body

Most of our thoughts, concepts and attitudes are learned in childhood, passed on from one generation to another from our family, school and culture. Prevailing views of right and wrong, and how to be healthy, are normally implied, sometimes strictly enforced, and it is human nature to keep on repeating, or reacting to, what we have been taught. One such cultural pattern is the belief that the body is like a machine and all we need to do is to take it to the doctor to get it fixed when something goes wrong.

Now studies show that there are other ways of perceiving health and addressing illness. It can take a long time for new research to be integrated into mainstream culture when it goes against well-established patterns. However the balance is shifting as scientific knowledge of quantum physics and studies of consciousness reveal the amazing effects of the mind on healing.[4]

WE CAN USE OUR MINDS IN WAYS WE NEVER DREAMED POSSIBLE

New research and open, scientifically rigorous and sustained discussions of all phenomena related to the mind offer new possibilities.[5] For example, Dr. Masaru Emoto, a Japanese scientist, became interested in how human consciousness affects the natural world. When he learned how to take photographs of the formation of natural frozen ice crystals, he discovered that under varying conditions major differences in crystal formation occur. Some were clearly shaped, others were deformed and, in some types of water, no crystals were formed at all. On a whim a colleague said, "Let's see what happens when we expose the water to music." They were amazed to find that water "listening to" classical music formed beautiful well-formed crystals while crystals exposed to violent heavy metal music resulted in fragmented and malformed crystals at best.

Thus started experiments that resulted in simple, vivid photography, demonstrating dramatically how molecules of water are affected by human thoughts, words and feelings.[6] Water also responded to the sentiment of words written on paper and placed around or underneath the water container. Written or spoken words like "Thank you" led to beautiful complete crystals, whereas chaotic thoughts or angry expressions like "You fool!" resulted in chaotic jagged shapes or no crystal formation at all. These findings held true, no matter the language used.

Since humans are largely composed of water, the implications of this for health are clear. We now have a chance to see for ourselves how consciousness affects everything, including things we previously thought of as inanimate or solid. Dr. Emoto's photographs can help us realize that wishes for peace, gratitude and love lead to a healthy response while blaming others or neglecting the self can subtly breed illness.

Healing Attitudes and Habits

When my heart is open, I flow easily through the day, resilient to all that life brings, in harmony with others and myself. And it's a great day to be alive! It's a different story when I feel out of sorts. If I have exhausted myself, I easily get into a flap in the face of all I have to do; or if something has gone wrong that displeases me or if my expectations have not been met, I become edgy and tense and all too soon I close my heart.

That's when I am likely to look for reasons outside myself to justify my negative feelings. However, I have learned that I have a choice in those moments. I can continue to feed my self-righteousness and fall into the trap of blaming others, or I can take time to discover and acknowledge my part in the situation and do the inner work of shifting and healing old patterns. I can explore how I'd really like to respond authentically in the troubling situation. I can take responsibility for living up to my own values rather than spiraling down into self-pity.

Below are some personal examples of changing old self-sabotaging attitudes and behaviors that hinder healing. Most are universally applicable, yet since each of our lives is so different, you will most likely have other attitudes you wish to release and affirmative thoughts you choose to welcome.

Letting Go of Judgment and Blame

It is tempting to latch onto a reason for your cancer and obsess about it, either judging yourself or blaming someone else, the environment, or God. I discovered I could ruminate on any number of reasons. Some or none of them might be real, for there are likely to be many contributing factors. Fixating on reasons is like grasping at straws in the wind. It drains your energy. Your primary job right now is to heal, so let go of being the critic, as much as you possibly can.

"No praise, no blame" is a very helpful attitude in which you put the filter of your judging mind aside in order to widen your attention and be in a place of open-ended inquiry. A judging mind makes things good or bad, right or wrong, according to a set of beliefs or dogma it has been trained to adhere to. The mind in this state is not able to be truly open to the present moment with its clues, messages and subtle nuances from sensations, fleeting memories, images or feelings. If you can be open to the moment, you may discover gifts within your illness. I found kindness at times when I least expected it—a phone call, a letter or a gift of homemade soup.

VALUING YOUR OWN CONTRIBUTION

Saying "yes" and "no" seems so straightforward, but it is sometimes difficult to do so. Many of us frequently say "yes" when we want to say "no," and "no" when we long to say "yes." Wanting to please and fearing disapproval, I grew up often playing it safe. I'd qualify an outer "yes" or "no" with an inner "if," "maybe" or "perhaps" loophole in my mind. Giving mixed signals is not a healthy state of affairs.

If you discover that you have been wobbling around saying this and that, hesitating to declare what you really think, stop! Take time to check in with yourself to discover what your honest opinion is before you say anything. If you are unsure, it's okay to say, "I'm not ready to give you an answer yet. I will get back to you." That way you will contribute more clearly to any conversation or decision when you are ready to speak. Since "yes" lets something in and "no" keeps something out, healthy boundaries are important. They inform people of where you and they stand; others don't have to second-guess you; and boundaries protect you from being in situations you sense will not be good for you.

EXPRESSING YOUR THANKFULNESS

From the rising of the sun, to the twinkling of the stars, give thanks!

A grateful attitude is of prime importance in all religious and indigenous traditions and is now underscored by Dr. Emoto's photography, as described in the previous chapter. From the rising of the sun, to the twinkling of the stars, give thanks! Let even the smallest flower on your path open your heart in love. Being appreciative changes a half empty glass to a half full one. Let your team know you don't take their contributions for granted. Smile at the office receptionist. Thank staff members you encounter for any courtesy, and be appreciative of the jobs they do. Some hospital workers may be doing low-paid, thankless tasks. Your attitude makes a difference.

As I was writing this last sentence, I remembered how appreciative I was, and am, for everyone involved with my surgery. The medical team worked together flawlessly. It was a remarkably nurturing day from beginning to end and I was very thankful for the skill and, yes, love of the hospital staff I experienced. I'm sorry now to admit that, although I expressed my thanks verbally, I didn't send a tangible expression, such as a card, to anyone at the time. If you are too overwhelmed to do so at the time, you can always do so later.

EMPOWERING LANGUAGE

Language matters. It helps to start sentences with words that empower and bring out the best in you such as "I choose," "I can," "I have" and "I love." If you use words that indicate you are a victim in some way, such as "I can't," "I need," "I'll try," or "I want," you will continue to manifest some form of lack or deficiency that prevents you from reaching your goal.

Provide your own answers to these questions, letting the examples trigger your own responses:

Discover and release your self-sabotaging attitudes and habits

- What actions do you wish to do differently? e.g. speak with less hesitation; listen before you speak.
- What old negative habits no longer serve you? e.g. criticizing others.
- What roles have you outgrown even though they once fulfilled you? e.g. being a caretaker of others but not yourself.
- What aspects of your life have you outgrown, but still keep doing out of habit? e.g. listening to others rather than your inner guidance.
- What do you secretly long to do, but don't let yourself do? e.g. change your work; learn photography; put your feet up and read a book.
- What thoughts undermine your wish to do something differently? e.g. self-doubt.

Discover and enhance your healing attitudes

- Think of people you admire. What qualities make each of them special?
- What qualities would you like to express in your own life?
- Finish this sentence: I am most contented when I am being _____ and/or _____.

- Practice saying "I choose ___," "I can___," "I have___" and "I love___."
- What attitudes support your healing?

3. If You Can Feel It, You Can Heal It—How Your Emotions Contribute to Healing

YOUR FEELINGS ARE IMPORTANT

A cancer journey can have many surprising twists and turns. At times you may feel as if you are on an emotional roller coaster. Don't minimize or underestimate the experience you are having. Take heart especially if your head is spinning and your emotions are bursting at the seams. Feelings of doubt, inadequacy, fear and anger are natural. In fact, your feelings *can* guide you. Listen for those feelings of discomfort. They may alert you to something you need to be cautious about or to examine further. On the other hand, if you feel comfortable or good about a specific situation, you are likely to be receiving an affirmative message, a green light to go forward in that direction.

You may experience more than one strong feeling, even contradictory ones at the same time, especially but not only in the early days of hearing your diagnosis. This is quite normal. You may be scared about what is ahead one moment, angry or even furious that you have cancer the next moment, and soon after that you may want to run away and ignore it all. It's important to acknowledge shock and to express your feelings—whatever they are—at your loss of health.

Feelings that are likely to surface when you are grieving have been identified. In fact, there are typical responses normally present in any kind of change bringing loss, be it relocation, retirement, loss of health or death of a loved one.[7] You are not alone if you want to deny that you have cancer, are angry or resentful about it, perhaps want to bargain your way out of it or get depressed.

Be aware that, although disconcerting, it is good for you to bring all these feelings to the light of day, in order for them to be addressed and healed. Belleruth Naparstek, author of *Staying Well with Guided Imagery,* calls this a "natural kind of rinsing." What is happening in your life is new. You have never been in this exact situation before. Witnessing, releasing and reframing your feelings can promote healing. It often helps to share these feelings with a trusted family member, friend or counselor.

FACING FEAR

Under normal circumstances, we're all angry and fearful from time to time. When a person is diagnosed with cancer, fears erupt all over the place—fear about making the wrong treatment decision, of pain, of possible treatment side effects, of a re-occurrence and of death. All become magnified. So much fear surrounds cancer in our medical establishments and in our culture at large that it rubs off on us all.

So much fear surrounds cancer in our medical establishments and in our culture at large that it rubs off on us all.

Following the shock of my diagnosis, I began to notice how I felt more fear immediately after some doctor visits, or after talking to someone who expressed their fears about my condition. I didn't want my treatment decisions to be driven by fear. Nor did I want to pretend my fears weren't there. When I was in touch with my fear or noticed I was absorbing fear from others, I began to be persistent in using self-care techniques—over and over again.

For example, I found it useful to take some deep slow breaths and then pay attention to my feet so that I could feel myself standing firmly on the ground. According to indigenous Senoi teachings, feelings in dreams contain messages within them and fear is the specific feeling that can lead us to our power, if we face it. They say, "Fear is an arrow pointing to power." When I am afraid I remember that and I ask myself, "How do I need to empower myself in this situation?" or "How can I gather the courage to face an upcoming appointment?" and even at times, "How can I best prepare for death?"

USING THE MESSAGE OF ANGER CONSTRUCTIVELY

Anger can be a very hot, uncomfortable emotion and many of us who were trained to be "good" find it easier to keep our anger to ourselves. When I am angry, I again feel my feet on the ground and breathe deeply into my stomach. I visualize sending my excess anger down through my legs and feet to be composted in the earth or I shake it off my hands. Then, since anger usually lets me know that some sort of change is needed, I ask myself some of these questions—"What is the message of my anger?" "How can I change, or what do I want to change?" "Have I been bottling up my feelings and swallowing back what I want to say?" "How might I express my needs, boundaries and feelings more directly?" or "How might I take care of myself now before my feelings build up even more and explode unexpectedly and inappropriately?"

If we hide anger away for a very long time, it can turn into a chilling bitterness and resentment. Such emotions stress the immune system.

If we hide anger away for a very long time, it can turn into a chilling bitterness and resentment. Such emotions stress the immune system. Once in cold storage, they lose heat and immediacy but they are not dead. When I notice I am resentful, I am reminded of Robert Burns' poem Tam O' Shanter in which Tam's wife sits at home "nursing her wrath to keep it warm." It seems pertinent to ask myself, "Have I been nurturing others but not myself?" and "How have I been harboring and feeding my grudges?"

CATCHING YOUR DREAMS

Dreams were used in the ancient world for both diagnosis and treatment. A well-respected tool, a dream was thought to provide the key for treatment. Shamans in some cultures would enter the dream state on the ill person's behalf to ask for guidance for how to proceed with healing. Your dreams are a message from your inner self.

Everything in your dreams is your creation. This is good news since you can use the material in your dreams to get a sense of your latent feelings—especially those that you are not quite aware of just beneath the surface. Your dreams may be about your interactions with others. Or they may reveal parts of yourself that you have been ignoring in daily life or that are struggling, fighting or yearning to be integrated. Your dreams often speak indirectly and subtly in symbols, images, sights, sounds, tastes and smells. Thus, dreams of death are not necessarily to be taken literally. They are much more likely to be telling you symbolically that something within you is dying, or expressing a fear. Just as in the fall trees shed their leaves at the end of the season, so too you may be entering a season where you must let go of the old so that something new may grow. Respect your dreams.

- Before you fully awaken and other thoughts intrude, lie quietly to become aware of whether you have been dreaming. If possible, don't use an alarm clock to jolt you out of sleep; try to linger in the half-sleep, half-awake state to get the feeling of your dream. That way you may catch a dream by its tail and remember more.
- Immediately thereafter, before you get up, write down whatever you remember in your journal for later exploration or speak it into a recording device.
- Retell the dream to yourself in the present tense as if it is happening now. This will give you a clearer sense of the immediacy and the feeling tone of the dream.
- Be on the lookout for any puns or play on words, and any symbols or people who might represent parts of yourself. This may give you clues about an issue you are now facing or feelings you may choose to heal.

Dreams sometimes reveal meaning through a play on words, as in this dream fragment: "A friend and I were looking out from a café. We saw three huge bears walking down the opposite side of the street on their hind legs beside people who didn't seem to notice them. We went out of the café to get a better look. The bears saw us and we became quite frightened. We sensed they were coming over to our cafe for lunch—which might be us! One bear grabbed my leather pocketbook, but we got safely inside and shut the door." In working with the dream I began to recognize how vulnerable and apprehensive I become when I share my inner feelings (bare my soul), and how I need to be more assertive like a bear (but not over-bearing) in expressing my truth or going for what I need. The resolution isn't in swinging from one extreme to the other, expressing anger or hiding it, but in developing a mature and balanced confidence to express myself clearly and appropriately.

Getting Help From a Psychotherapist May Be Wise

If feelings about your diagnosis are overwhelming you, your family or your support circle, don't hesitate to go to a counselor or therapist. The seeds of dis-ease that lead to illness may have been lying dormant for many years. One person who is an over-active caretaker of others might find she has been harboring a grudge about how much she has been taken for granted. Another might uncover a hurt or angry, neglected "inner child" who wants love.

More importantly, as a cancer patient, look for a therapist who will focus on what is right with you and will help you discover and make decisions that will lead you to living your kind of life, one that makes you glad to wake up in the morning. Research from many countries shows that this approach, no matter the stage of cancer, will help mobilize self-healing abilities and bring them to the aid of your medical program. While wonderfully effective in other situations, focusing on "What is wrong with you?" and "How did you get that way?" does not work well for cancer patients.[8]

In therapy or counseling, the therapeutic relationship is itself a powerful part of the process of healing. A trained counselor should not be upset with anything you say, whereas those close to you, who are dealing with their own feelings about your cancer, might be. In fact, it can be a relief to others to know that you have professional support. A therapist can help you deal with an over-abundance of feelings that are spilling out or help you thaw out feelings you may have put in deep freeze so that you didn't need to feel them. When life is too painful, it is wise to ask for help. In the presence of a counselor, you can safely allow your feelings to surface, find words to express them to others or to yourself, release them, forgive others or yourself, and make new choices. If you don't know what your feelings are, a therapist can also be very helpful. A body-oriented psychotherapist, combining emotional and physical work, might be of particular help.

- When new feelings surface, sense your feet firmly connected to the ground. Deepen and soften your breathing.
  - ~ Put your hand on your belly for comfort, or give yourself a hug; or ask for one.
  - ~ Give your negative feelings a color and drain them out of your body by sending the color down your legs into the ground to be absorbed and transformed by the earth. The earth is an expert at taking negativity (garbage which would make us sick) and turning it into compost for future healthy growth.

or

  - ~ Since we often forget that we can hold onto old negative feelings in our belly or in our heart for a very long time, imagine you are moving any such feelings of annoyance, irritation or anger from deep inside you. Move them first towards your extremities and then to the outside by literally shaking or flicking them off from your fingers, arms, legs and ankles.
- Take a shower and, as you clean your skin, ask the water to cleanse and purify your feelings. Let any tears of sadness flow with the water.
- Reach out to a friend.
- Choose some favorite music. Let the music nourish you and lead you into deeper comfort or greater relaxation.
- Use colored crayons or markers to draw a picture of how you feel in your journal. Perhaps shut your eyes or use your non-dominant hand and give permission for your hand to express itself, bypassing your rational mind with its judgments and expectations.

Actions to love and support yourself when strong feelings arise

WHATEVER YOU FEED GROWS LARGER; WHATEVER YOU STARVE SHRINKS

"Whatever you feed grows larger; whatever you neglect or starve shrinks" can be applied to everything you do. Every healthy choice builds a foundation for the next healthy choice. Every feeling you express contributes to who you are becoming in one way or another.

An old Indian warrior was talking with his grandson. He described a battle that goes on inside people. He said, "The battle that goes on is between two wolves. One is Evil. It is anger, envy, regret, greed, arrogance, self-pity, guilt, lies, false pride, superiority and ego. The other is Good. It is joy, peace, love, humility, kindness, empathy, generosity, truth, compassion and faith." The grandson thought for a while and asked, "Which wolf wins?" His grandfather replied simply, "The one you feed."

Esther   *I've found taking care of myself has been an opportunity to learn about all-embracing compassion, for myself, as well as others. Love, kindness and gratitude are attributes I can cultivate as a daily practice. This journey has brought me in direct contact with my deepest fears, and I've discovered that I have far more choice than I ever realized to direct and be in control of my feelings. I choose to let go of destructive attachments, indulging in "poor me" and putting too much emphasis on the future. I make it a practice to stay present and be grateful for every day on this good earth.*

What do you feed?

- What feelings do you wish to welcome and expand, as contributing to your health?
- What negative feelings have you been overindulging or emphasizing?
- List those feelings you wish to expand and those you wish to release in order to give more space for healing.
- Choose one action that will bring you joy—today.

4. From Sole to Soul—How Your Spirit Contributes to Healing

A number of years ago a friend told me how surprised she was when an oncologist, speaking to a group of cancer patients about treatment issues, added, "And if you don't have a spiritual life—get one!" It was the last thing she expected to hear since he was a doctor, not a priest, rabbi or imam. The oncologist explained his statement by referring to new research, which showed that spiritual practices contribute significantly to healing.

Does prayer, for example, really affect our healing? Until recently I would have said, "Yes, I am sure, but I can't prove it." Now I too can point to the affirmative results of many scientific experiments as well as my own experience. The rewards of consistent meditation and prayer are well documented. Scientific studies, described by Larry Dossey, MD,[9] and others who started out as skeptics, show that both have a very positive effect on healing in plants, animals and humans.

SPIRITUAL PRACTICES CAN HELP US HEAL

When cancer cuts into our lives, it challenges each of us in different ways. It upsets regular routines and demands different priorities. Yet it can awaken awareness of our spiritual nature, and take us from living on the surface of life to deeper experiences. No matter what is going on in your cancer journey, you can tap into resources beyond the physical, which can have a marked effect on the physical. Spiritual practices can open a door to deeply healing connections between yourself and the universe. Their beneficial results can be experienced in many ways—physical, emotional, and spiritual.

It doesn't seem to matter whether you already have a faith that brings comfort and strength or whether you have found organized religion to be too uncomfortable or whether you have simply turned away from spiritual matters. Spiritual practices do not belong to any one system or set of structures. They can work for us all, and under any circumstances. We can all attune our awareness, develop our attention and open our perceptions. Through taking time out for spiritual practices you affirm that you are more than just a patient defined by a cancer diagnosis. You can feed your soul, your connection with the mystery of life and your longing for healing.

The rewards of consistent meditation and prayer are well documented.

For example, some people think of prayer as communicating with a Universal Power—some Life Force or Intelligence beyond themselves to which or whom they can give thanks, and from which or whom they can ask for help and perhaps carry on problem-solving discussions—not always known as God.[10] All her life Marion Woodman's relationship to Sophia, a divine inner feminine wisdom presence, has sustained her, and so it was to Sophia that she turned before a radiation treatment: "Dear Sophia, please keep your shield over my belly and over my heart. Yes, over my eyes. I feel somewhat blind after the treatment. Please protect my skin. Please protect my bowels from being burned. Please protect me from human error. Fill me with ultraviolet light. Let me take on as much of the higher energies as possible without damage to my body. Thank you. Thank you for your love that forever upholds me."[11]

Students of Yoga, Chi Kung and Tai Chi often learn to meditate through movement and through sinking into the practice of watching the breath. Those who have a heartfelt connection to nature may pray by taking long walks or sitting with openness beside a waterfall. Dance and movement can also be a doorway to meditation. Music can be the same. Buddhists feel a deep calm resting in the basic goodness of life without reference to any external God. There are many other forms of spiritual practice—ranging from prayers around the kitchen table and blessing or healing ceremonies outdoors to kneeling, chanting, singing and bowing in places of worship. Each of these ways has enriched my life and comforted me at difficult times.

The broad spectrum of ways to enhance healing—relaxation, music, art, movement, connecting to nature, doing what you love and journal-writing—can all be used to deepen your understanding and connection to the presence of God or The Divine. So too can the work of transforming your negative thoughts and emotions into life-giving affirmations described in the previous sections. A spiritual practice can be born out of intention. You can invent one.

I have come to know that any activity, even everyday tasks including my cancer appointments, can become a spiritual practice, when done with love and awareness.

HOW TO NURTURE YOUR SPIRITUAL LIFE WHEN YOU HAVE CANCER

Here is a selection of a limited number of well-tested spiritual practices involving prayer and meditation that I found to be healing. Many encourage silence and letting go into a deeper way of being. Being quiet is especially valuable when worry or distress knocks repeatedly at the door.

Consider before you begin—

- It is beneficial to set aside daily times to establish regularity. Most people suggest morning and/or evening.
- The practices you embark on need not be elaborate. Initially, it is better to commit to a shorter, simple "discipline" than a longer one. You can start with about 10 minutes of quiet time. When you are comfortable with short periods, lengthen the time you spend.
- It is often recommended that you do such practices on an empty stomach or after a light snack, not immediately after a heavy meal.
- Use your intuition to guide you to the practices that resonate with you.

- Treatment regimes will affect what you are able to do. Days of bed-rest are very different from days when you are combining a work schedule with treatment. Sometimes your spiritual practices may be minimal. At other times, you may be able to extend them.
- "Early birds" and "night owls" will probably be wise to take into account their different biorhythms when deciding the best time to explore a practice. Most practices can be done at any time—morning, noon or night.

Don't just do something, sit there!

Try one of the following quiet ways of praying and meditating

- Sit with your eyes closed. Begin to contemplate the amazing miracle of life. Be receptive and open to whatever comes.
- If you wish to be more focused, fill your mind quietly with thoughts of a quality like truth, beauty, love, grace, or awareness of the blessings in your life. Sense it in your body.
- After listening to a quiet guided imagery audio or piece of music linger in a meditative or prayerful attitude.

Count your breath

The practice of counting the breath is an ancient meditative practice, used for centuries to clear the mind, silence thoughts and develop relaxation.

- Focus only on one thing, namely counting your breath. Breathe in, then as you breathe out, say silently "one"; breathe in again and on the out-breath say silently, "two," and so on: in—out, "three," in—out, "four." Keep repeating this simple cycle of counting one to four. Whenever your thoughts wander to something else, gently bring them back to counting your breath again. I found this strange when I was first introduced to it, but I grew to like its simplicity.

Walk quietly

The act of walking while you are meditating, allows you to discharge excess energy so that as you focus inwards you become like a clear bell or an unruffled pool of water.

- On any walk, let your gaze soften just in front of you and become very aware of every step you take, step by step by step.
- Stop at any peaceful place from time to time.
- Notice Mother Nature's exquisite detail—a tiny flower, a robin's egg, a fallen feather—or her vast vistas after rounding a curve. Perhaps you'll absorb the silence or listen to the birds. Her gifts are everywhere, leading you to gratitude and meditation.
- As you walk, ask an inner question regarding a current issue in your life. Tune in to any message that comes to you about your life and health.

USE PRAYERFUL WORDS

- Ask for healing in whatever way is best for you.
- As you pray for healing, visualize yourself well and happy, rather than focusing on a specific problem.
- If at the beginning you find it hard to pray for yourself, you might want to encourage or allow others to do so on your behalf—the more the better!
- Give your name to a local healing or prayer circle.
- Call a prayer hotline, such as Unity at 816-NOW-PRAY (1-800-669-7729). I have found their volunteers to be extremely skilled and understanding. A volunteer will ask you, "How may we pray with you?" He/she listens to what you reply and then offers a prayer while you are on the phone. (International callers: use 1-816 969-2000).
- Listen to, or join in singing along with, music that resonates with your core, such as African American gospel songs, "Fiddler on the Roof," or hymns and songs of your youth, if that brings comfort or joy.
- Memorize several short passages of scripture or poetry so that you can hold on to one by repeating it to yourself like an affirmation when you are agitated, for example, while waiting for treatment.

EXPLORE SPIRITUAL READINGS

- Use one of the many daily guides such as *The Daily Word*, *Meditations for Women Who Do Too Much*, or *Science of*

Mind. The simple structure of one page at a time for one day at a time—with a quote from an inspiring text or a wise person, followed by a brief commentary on the theme for daily prayer or affirmation, is easy to follow.

- Read from poets and mystics such as Mary Oliver, T. S. Eliot, Nancy Wood, Rumi or Hafiz to enrich and feed your soul. If you read a poem several times, you may discover and absorb different layers.

- Select a sequence of passages directly from the Bible, the Koran or other sacred texts.

- You might "google" for daily meditations sites with quotes and calming images or go to www.beliefnet.com for their daily inspiration and/or daily prayer. Whatever you hold in reverence can be your "Holy Scriptures."

- Starting the day in one of these ways can prepare you beautifully to listen to a meditation audio, do yoga stretches, sit in silence or do one of the things you might select for your own wellness program after reading Chapter 7.

HELP ON YOUR SPIRITUAL PATH

Spiritual counseling or mentoring

Just as some people go to a therapist for help with emotional issues, you can seek support from a professional spiritual or pastoral counselor or a volunteer/lay spiritual mentor. Expect this person to affirm you as you share your searching and doubts as well as your faith and trust. This can be of great help when facing the "dark night of the soul," when life painfully cuts deep into your core. As in nature, the darkest time is often just before the dawn, which can be the very moment you are tempted to give up. That's when you need encouragement to hang in there.

- If you already are part of a church, synagogue, mosque or other community, you may want to turn to someone you already know and trust to be a mentor, or ask them for professional referrals.

- If you don't belong to any institutional belief system, look for someone who respects your spiritual journey and who will listen to you without diverting you or telling you what to believe. You may find such a person through your professional contacts or by word of mouth. Perhaps you can find someone who has walked in your shoes as a cancer patient.

- Once you have identified a possible spiritual mentor, create an opportunity to have an open-ended conversation with that person to see if you are both comfortable talking about the things that matter to you. If you value the views and support expressed and it feels right to you, request further conversations. If not, look for another person.

- If you feel an intuitive pull to connect with a living spiritual teacher (e.g. The Dalai Lama, Marianne Williamson, Thich Nhat Hanh, Pema Chodron, or Eckhart Tolle), read their books, listen to a video or go to a conference where they are speaking. This too can support healing.

Group support

Without support and encouragement of others, it is easy to neglect spiritual aspects of life. If you feel isolated in your inner quest or if your family is discouraging, you may find it especially helpful to re-connect with a spiritual or religious group or community. It can help rekindle your trust and faith in life. If your spiritual perspectives have changed, trust your need to seek out a new group that is in line with who you are now.

Inner support

Without even traveling from your house or bed, you can get support from people you admire. When you need comfort, you might remember a loving grandparent and imagine what he or she might say to you. When you need courage, you might call to mind strong figures like Martin Luther King or Helen Keller. Let their written or spoken words inspire you, or read about them. Whether they are close or far, alive or from centuries ago doesn't matter. What happens in your inner world is up to you.

- Sit quietly and have a silent conversation with a person you admire. Invite their help and support for general healing or for a specific situation.[12]

Esther The most important factor in my healing has been putting my spiritual practice back into a primary position. In retrospect I realize I slowly had become more and more concerned about the state of the world, listening more frequently to politically-oriented material and reducing my spiritual practices. I reversed this, putting meditation, appreciation, being in the present moment as the most important components in my life. I still am active politically but I do not start off my day listening to the world. Instead I tune into what inspires me, whether music, singing, sitting, praying, sending healing energy or focusing on beauty. After the tone of my day is set I will then selectively allow the news to come in. I still can be affected by one horror story after another. Knowing the immune system is weakened by stress, worry and fear, I make it a practice to stay focused on what I love, desire and what inspires me. I notice if my mind moves into the old habit of focusing on what I don't want, and then I gently redirect it.

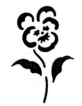

9

Quests, Questions, Mysteries and Miracles

MANY PEOPLE WHO HAVE LITTLE OR NO RELATIONSHIP to their depths when they are physically fit suddenly find themselves praying or asking profound questions when they become ill. Cancer can challenge you to dig deeper to uncover or return to a more meaningful sense of your place in the world.

THE MYSTERY OF CANCER'S WAKE-UP CALL

Part of the magnificence of human beings is that we can constantly renew ourselves, from the tiniest cell to the largest muscle or bone. Yet it is frequently a mystery why this life-giving capacity fails to prevent cancer in people who actively maintain their health. There are no easy equations. A positive attitude will not necessarily cure you, nor will a "bad" attitude necessarily kill you.

Whether you believe your illness is entirely caused by environmental or genetic factors beyond your control, or not, you can choose to let cancer be a wake-up call to wellness. It may mean throwing out toxic chemical cleaning products, paying special attention to diet, clearing out old emotional baggage, perhaps finding forgiveness for an old wound or nurturing your spiritual life.

Cancer is also likely to bring you face to face with questions that slip through in unguarded moments, questions about life, *your* life and death, your strength and fragility.

QUESTIONS, QUESTIONS, QUESTIONS

When you are diagnosed, you may start out with practical questions—

- What treatment should I opt for?
- Who will take care of me?

Then you might ask—

- Why didn't I know a long time ago that something was wrong?

Deeper spiritual questions may follow—

- Why me?
- Who am I?
- Is there a purpose for this experience of cancer? And if so, what?
- Is there a God? Or who or what is my God?

Leading to—

- How do I really want to live?
- What regrets do I have?
- To whom do I need to apologize? Whom do I need to forgive?
- What if this is it—the beginning of the end?
- Am I ready to die?
- Is there a part of me that does not start with birth and does not end with death?

Many questions are layered, with one answer on the surface and another underneath. Going deeper takes tremendous courage. Most of us feel vulnerable when we speak of our inner uncertainties. There are a number of reasons for this. We have learned along the way that such conversations are all too often taboo. We don't want our fragile, tentative thoughts and feelings to be trampled on. And we don't have the language to talk about experiences that can take us beyond rational understanding.

Yet through the challenge of cancer's darkest moments, we may find answers to our innermost longings. Heartfelt questioning can become like a Zen koan, which in Eastern traditions is a puzzle that cannot be answered logically but pursuing it can lead to new awareness.

LIFE IN DEATH, DEATH IN LIFE

When I was beginning to write this chapter, on the spur of the moment, I listened to a PBS television program that touched me profoundly. It was billed as "One Man's Journey" (through the Canadian wilderness.)[1] I had no inkling that woven throughout would be a story of how this man's partner, Irene, struggled with cancer. Irene spoke simply of her worst times of despair and how she never before knew how deep into herself she could go on this journey "she would never have chosen in a million years." She talked of how she lived with the unknown, not knowing whether she would live or die and how she feared death and was not ready to say goodbye to those whom she loved.

When she and her beloved Robert knew her death was coming closer she said, "Don't worry, I'll be around. You can't fall out of the universe."

In her mind's eye, Irene saw a little delicate flower pushing its way up through the concrete. She wanted to pounce on it, but she knew if she grabbed it she would kill it. She decided she would just have to watch it and honor it, this tiny fragile flower. It was perhaps a metaphor for her life. She began to have less fear about her eventual death and later, she saw all of life, including death, as a continuum. The hardest part, she said, was trying to understand why she became sick at such an early age. Recognizing that there may not be an answer, she learned to live with the unknowable. When she and her beloved Robert knew her death was coming closer she said, "Don't worry, I'll be around. You can't fall out of the universe."

This young woman's simple acceptance of her imminent death remained with me. The phrase "You can't fall out of the universe" kept reverberating in my head. I delved deeper into my own understandings of death as I asked myself, "What did she mean?" I felt I had been given a tiny flower to treasure in my inner world and to pass on to you. Here was a woman who had courageously risked asking the deepest questions. I felt she asked them for me and I was blessed to experience her spirit shining through the television program.

The "C" word (cancer) and the "D" word (death), unmentionable by many, are both linked to fear. Yet there are many kinds of death—of old cells, old ways, old beliefs, and old relationships. In the course of our life, we may die many times. It's beneficial to look at death on many levels. For all of us, at some point, death will come to the physical body.

Yet symbolic figures of death, for example in dreams, are often actually announcing that it is time to let part of life die so that something new can be born in its place. The card named *Death* in the traditional tarot is a good example. It stirs fear but it actually indicates rebirth. When you are able to confront and even befriend your fears, they may reveal that you are ready for something new. Perhaps you have become strong enough to release an aspect of yourself that you have been desperately clinging to, or to see things in a different light. When you struggle against these intimations, deny or block them out, they are more likely to become a source of terror, sometimes surfacing in your dreams.

When you are able to confront and even befriend your fears, they may reveal that you are ready for something new.

In contrast to Irene, Meg consciously pushed her fears of change and death away. As long as she tried to ignore them, she was stalked by a dark, cloaked figure in her dreams. When she sought help to engage with this presence and explore what he might want to say to her, her dreams took a new shape. She understood that part of her life was indeed dying and it was futile to pretend otherwise. Every now and then, if she ignored what the figure had indicated to her, he reappeared in her dreams.

CHALLENGES TO SHAKE UP THE SOUL

"To every thing there is a season and a time to every purpose under heaven...a time to be born, and a time to die; a time to plant, and a time to pluck up that which is planted; a time to kill and a time to heal."[2] Life brings to each human being a full palette of experiences. As well as times of light and joy, there are winter storms when you are tested to the limits and life is experienced as unforgiving and painfully raw. If, through cancer, you enter the "dark night of the soul," as it is called in most spiritual traditions, you have not been personally targeted or punished, although it may feel like that. The experiences you would never choose for yourself are part of life's deepest mystery.

An old story tells of a farmer who thought he would teach God a thing or two about farming. He asked God to let him be in charge. He knew he could grow a bumper crop and then there would be no more poverty. God agreed to give him a year to put his plan into action, and everything the farmer asked for was granted—no thunder, no strong winds or dangers for the crops; only sun and rain when he wanted them. The crops grew high and the farmer said, "See, there will be enough wheat for 10 years!" The wheat grew even higher, but when it was harvested, he was shocked to find there was no wheat inside. He asked God what went wrong, and God said, "Because there was no challenge, because there was no conflict, no friction, because you avoided all that was bad, the wheat remained impotent... A little struggle is a must. Storms are needed, thunder, lightning is needed. They shake up the soul inside the wheat."[3]

Cancer can challenge you to painstakingly weed out mutating cells and, perhaps, parts of your life that you have unconsciously hosted for years. There is a time to uproot, a time to heal—and then for all of us—a time to die, some sooner, some later.

Cancer can carve out your being, making you more whole through the hurts, sadness and suffering that you experience.

THE MYSTERY OF "GOD"

The word God, like the word love, has so many meanings that it has become a confusing term. While some people are very comfortable with God, others are not. They prefer a different name and language for what was traditionally known as God, Hashem, Allah or Great Spirit. The Divine is not easily defined and spiritual teachers through the centuries have reminded us that whatever name we use is not "It."

Puja In my childhood I was taught that this greater reality or Higher Power was named God, definitely a masculine being, separate and beyond us. Through a widening circle of experience, I became aware of the feminine face of God and later a Divine Presence, a Creative Process or Life Force within me and throughout all life. I prefer to be inclusive.

It doesn't ultimately seem to matter what we call God or even if we use that word at all. Whatever your definition, it is healthy to allow room for new understandings and nuances, for "It" cannot be explained or contained in language anyway.

MIRACULOUS MOMENTS

I believe there is a great mystery connecting all of life. Although our technological society has elevated rational logical thinking at the expense of intuition, I'm glad life's mystery has never faded. I'm among those who experience a sense of wonder at the intricacies of the universe and our place in it.

When Sondra Barrett was researching leukemia, she used the microscope to study human blood cells. "It was like watching a magical mystery unfold," she wrote. The vitamin B12 looked like outer space! Her "a-ha" moment, through witnessing the miraculous beauty of science, inspired her to give slide shows to children with cancer. These children and, later, adults were amazed to see sick cells, healthy cells and the many chemicals that made up the secret drama of life and death in their own bodies. Later she apprenticed to a shaman, and learned how to look beyond the visible. She could sense that the tiny cells were enfolded with divine wisdom and were teachers of how to live a sacred life; and this she could pass on.[4]

Since life is not logical or linear, the unexpected is always round the corner. Moments of surprising joy and healing come in spite of sadness. You may have experienced a sudden unsought awakening to a hitherto unknown dimension, or an unexpected life-changing experience that turned everything that you'd believed upside down. Perhaps you had a miraculous healing. Maybe you've felt overwhelming gratitude and love during an ordinary day, or wonder and awe at the beauty of nature has taken your breath away. While you cannot plan or grab those miraculous moments, you can be open to the possibility. I've certainly had my share of experiences for which I had no explanation, such as an awareness of protection in a near accident and a chance meeting with someone against all the odds. Such times of synchronicity or awareness of spiritual presence can be healing.

MIRACULOUS HEALINGS

Over the centuries, those searching for cures for serious illnesses have gathered at ancient healing waters and wells or at sites where miracles are said to have happened. Currently people still go to locations such as Lourdes in France hoping for miraculous cures—as well as to healers such as John of God in Brazil[5] or indigenous shamans on several continents, especially if they have not found, or choose not to find, all the answers within mainstream medicine.

I'm glad life's mystery has never faded. I'm among those who experience a sense of wonder at the intricacies of the universe and our place in it.

Many cancer patients, who travel long distances in their search for healing, do so as an expression of faith. Some come back miraculously cured or healed, while others do not. It is part of the mystery that there are no hard and fast guarantees, but certainly hope and faith each play a part in making healing possible. Never think of yourself as a cancer "victim," for such consciousness leads to feelings of helplessness and hopelessness that in turn can contribute to the disease process. You can change your perspectives and your energy. Deepak Chopra has suggested you can be fascinated with wellness rather than with illness and disease. He affirms that this one little shift can have great consequences. Some studies of neurotransmitters indicate that the physiology of hope can support healing. Follow your own sense of what you trust to bring the miracle of healing closer—it could be Western medicine, or some little known complementary option, or a combination of both.

As a consequence of studying hands-on healing and energy work with Rosalyn L. Bruyere,[6] taking other seminars,[7] and practicing as a therapist—all for decades, I've had numerous experiences that led me to know, deep within my being, the miraculous power of prayer and "laying-on-of-hands" healing both for myself and others.

Puja   *Once, when a team of colleagues was exploring the use of a specific energy technique with me, I described my concern about the texture I had been feeling up and down my inner left breast. It was lumpy like a rope and as they sent energy to the area, the image came to me of an old Gothic stone arch. After they completed the healing, the lumpiness was absolutely gone.*

Medical professionals often call such healings spontaneous remissions, if they don't have other ways of accounting for the phenomena. I prefer to acknowledge the energy source that we can plug into and receive, and I choose to give thanks to the Divine.

Never limit yourself by the fear and tyranny of statistics when a prognosis for your type of cancer is given. There is always more than meets the eye in any situation. No matter what diagnosis the doctors have given you, be open to the possibility of healing and contribute to it.

John was diagnosed with an inoperable brain tumor. His wife put out a desperate call for research of options and other help. His friends rallied round to search for any glimmer of hope. They sent emails with information and suggestions of this treatment and that, so much so that John was quite overwhelmed even after someone stepped in to edit them. Eventually a prayer circle was set up and three very experienced Reiki practitioners, two on the East coast (one being my friend who had faced his own cancer) and one on the West coast, coordinated a long distance healing session with John. At the time of the healing John knew something had shifted. Indeed it had. The headaches were gone and, as far as his doctors can tell, the cancer was in remission.

It will be easier if you see yourself as fluid rather than fixed or solid. From your first breath, till your last, you are riding a wave of energy that flows through, constantly animating and changing you. As Norman Brown says in *Love's Body*, "The human body is not a thing or a substance given, but a continuous creation. The human body is an energy system, which is never a complete structure, never static; it is in perpetual self-construction, self-destruction. We destruct in order to make it new." [8]

You can stimulate your "life force" to activate your body's own pharmacy (chemicals we make ourselves) to support healing. There are many ways to do this. For example, massage, reflexology, energy work, visualization and exercising will all help amplify other treatments you have, including medical treatments. Receiving hands-on-healing energy work, for example, helps to raise the energy level so that your basic vibration is higher than that of the low-frequency malignancy within you. [9]

To patients who are not familiar with this way of thinking, such healing may seem to be miraculous. Yet it can be explained in the terms and language of energy. Other patients marvel at what Western medicine can do. To them that is truly miraculous. We each have frontiers of knowledge—that we have come to know through training or experience, and that we don't know but which, through further study and experience, may be revealed. I believe that part of the mystery is that there will always be the unexplainable—and the unknowable.

It will be easier if you see yourself as fluid rather than fixed or solid. From your first breath, till your last, you are riding a wave of energy that flows through, constantly animating and changing you.

10 ❀

Ancient Pathways
to Healing

NCIENT SYSTEMS OF HEALING FROM THE EAST, SUCH
as Chinese medicine and Ayurveda, are becoming
popular in the west. Ordinary people are willing to
pay out of pocket for these services, and even grocery stores
regularly stock token organic and whole-food sections related
to these healing systems. It is clear that growing numbers of
people are taking charge of their health. Our perceptions of
how to maintain health are changing.

Personal choice and participation are also crucial to many
cancer patients who welcome what Western medicine has
to offer. These patients research all possible options, listen to
their inner voice and then embark on a healing program, selecting from both mainstream and complementary sources.
Here are examples of ancient pathways to healing, adapted
by patients for their current lifestyles and specific healing cri-
ses.

1. Healing Retreats

Marie, Jan, Tona and Kathy all chose to go to a residential
healing retreat. Here are their stories.

Marie When cancer struck, Marie started her quest for
healing by spending a month away from home boost-
ing her immune system at a health clinic in Florida. She rented a

condo and each week her husband, her daughter or a friend took time off to be with her.

Jan   Jan chose another path. She went to a retreat in California specially designed for cancer patients where a trained staff guided her, both medically and spiritually. The staff took into account who she was as a person, as they discussed possible treatments from a holistic perspective. Her search for spiritual meaning was acknowledged. That and her interaction with other participants became very important parts of the experience. Such retreat centers provide structure, integrated knowledge, support and companionship.[1]

Tona   Towards the end of her treatment, Tona found great encouragement in going to a conference in Vermont for cancer survivors that had some "retreat-like" aspects such as yoga classes and a rock-climbing wall. Local hotels donate rooms for this annual event. Tona had previously made a good connection with one of the organizers, a physician, and they had spoken on the phone a number of times. This association was very important to Tona especially because she knew that this doctor's tumor had been as big as her own, and that she had been living for nine years thus far after having had a late stage 3 diagnosis. More recently Tona chose to go on a retreat that had nothing directly to do with cancer but which she feels was very healing.

Kathy   Kathy was not aware, growing up, that she was a "DES Daughter" the term given to women exposed to DES, or diethylstilbestrol, in utero.[2] Intuitively she had been very particular about avoiding drugs of all kinds, even painkillers. Within a week of her diagnosis, she had been rushed into surgery. At the time, she felt privileged to have such swift attention. She then had a course of chemotherapy and radiation. Many months later, when the doctors discovered the cancer was not contained, she was offered more radiation. The doctors advised her husband that he should take six months off work and spend it with his family—since Kathy didn't have much more time than that to live. For Kathy, it was almost a freeing pronouncement. It meant that she had given the "conventional" treatment every opportunity, even though she had begun to suspect that it was now poisoning her. She wanted to try it her way. She took more time to think about her options. In spite of her doctors' doubts, she decided to go on an intensive course of cleansing at a residential retreat run by spiritually-oriented naturopathic doctors in Colorado. Kathy also wanted to learn how to balance her body when she returned home. The program included

She knows that the physical outcome is not guaranteed but the retreat brought hope and much comfort to Kathy, her husband and her two young children.

fasting and juicing as well as prayer, meditation and silence. She knows that the physical outcome is not guaranteed but the retreat brought hope and much comfort to Kathy and her family. Today, having followed the protocols for over a year, she is alive and has learned to live every moment in the now as a gift. She knows that healing is not just about curing the body.

Just as animals retreat to lick their wounds, you too, by retreating at times of illness, can aid your body's recuperative powers. This has been known and practiced for centuries. In fact had Marie, Jan, Tona, and Kathy lived in ancient Egypt or Greece, they might have spent time in a healing temple, the respected and conventional place for healing of that day.

Nowadays, some cancer patients choose to go on a day retreat, a silent retreat, a women's or men's retreat as part of their wellness program. Others create their own mini-retreat.

Puja   *Several years before my cancer, a friend gave me cassettes of the monks of Weston Priory in Vermont singing songs of faith. Their harmonious music was so comforting and inspiring that I played it time and again when driving. Before my surgery, I decided to attend services with the singing monks and spend time in their peaceful priory grounds. I found a local bed and breakfast in the vicinity where I could give myself a more leisurely start to the day and where I could be pampered with excellent food—just the right combination. The retreat helped me to connect to myself in a fundamental way so that I could return home refreshed for what was ahead.*

Imagine yourself on retreat

- What kind of healing retreat are you longing for?
- Are you in need of time away from your usual surroundings? Peace and quiet? Companionship? Solitude? Or something else_____?
- How long would you like your retreat to last?
- What practicalities need to be put in place? Who could help?
- Search the Internet for the type of retreat you wish or for other ideas.

2. The Healing Power of Community

I have taken part in many different kinds of healing circles, both for others and for myself. These ranged from those that came together only once to those that met regularly for quite a long time.

Before she started chemotherapy, Ujjala asked to have a healing circle with friends and family.

Ujjala *The blessings, support and gifts of love that came out of this healing circle gave me such strength and opened my eyes to the importance of receiving. It became a strong foundation for eight months of treatment ahead. I continued to ask to be on prayer lists and prayer circles, and to have spiritual energy healings from friends and small healing groups for the duration of my treatments.*

Five years later with a recurrence of cancer, when she found out how expensive her choice of complementary and alternative treatments was going to be, her community rallied round again. By organizing a dance celebration, they raised enough money for Ujjala to do her preferred treatments for a year. "The fact that people again gave to me so generously was another healing in itself," she said.

If you choose to invite trusted friends or family members to form a circle with you in your home or theirs, here are some well-tried suggestions for participation. It is helpful to have a unifying intention and focus for the gathering. Some circles come together to give practical and moral support in whatever ways they are requested. Others have traditionally shared prayers, readings, heartfelt words, music, or offered healing.

Imagine how you would like to involve loved ones in a healing circle

- What kind of circle would you like—one in which people are present with you? Or pray for you at a distance? Or both? If others are with you, where would you be—in the middle or part of the ring?

How to create a circle

- What would you wish the intention and focus for the gathering to be?
- Who would you invite to participate?
- Create a Facebook group for a cancer patient which friends and family are invited to join. Caringbridge.org and lotsa-helpinghands.com are also great ways to share information and coordinate requests for meals, rides, visits, etc.

Here are some options:

- Either take your place in the circle's ring or place yourself in the middle encircled by those invited to be present.
- Ask participants to form a "talking stick" circle in which the person holding the "stick" or other object talks from the heart, uninterrupted until he or she is ready to pass on the stick to another. The "stick" can circle round more than once, but there is no general conversation until the end of the circle.
- After you share your feelings and concerns, welcome love and understanding by inviting each person to speak to you from the heart. You may also ask for practical support.
- Ask those around you to turn to you with their palms open towards your body to convey healing energy as you sit in a chair or lie down. This can be done without actually touching you. If you welcome comfort from physical touch, invite your circle to place their hands gently on different parts of your body such as hands, shoulders, and feet. Let their hands rest there as they pass along love and healing to you. If you have friends who are trained in a specific healing modality such as Reiki, ask them to form a healing circle team. It is wonderful to receive such shared energy.
- If you feel shy or unsafe about having a circle, ask your family and friends to form an "invisible circle" around you—one in which, at an agreed time, they can tune in and send you loving energy from wherever they are.
- Ask your loved ones to form a prayer chain, where members pass on from person to person your request for prayer—and any other information you may wish to share with them.

3. Healing Pilgrimages

In my childhood a motley crew of Chaucer's Canterbury Pilgrims looked down from a painting above the mantelpiece in the living room. They were obviously having a good time![3] Thus began my fascination for pilgrimages. As a teenager, my first day-long pilgrimage took place on Iona, St. Columba's sacred isle, off the West coast of Scotland. Historically this island has been a place both of ancient energies and new beginnings.

A pilgrimage is an inward venture, taking place within an outer adventure. It can be a journey of faith, transforming ordinary travel plans into a personal quest—a tailor-made adventure that echoes what each person is seeking or holds reverently in their heart. A pilgrimage starts with longings, dreams, intentions and preparations—usually well before pilgrims set foot outside their doors. Thereafter follows the journey itself, the arrival at the destination, and finally the return back home. Your yearning for healing might call you to go with others or alone, in the spirit of a pilgrimage, to a far distant sacred site. Or you could equally well make your way to a local park, a forest, botanical gardens, or to the edge of the ocean.

A pilgrimage is an inward venture, taking place within an outer adventure.

Puja   As an adult, before my cancer experience, I had my own tradition of making a personal pilgrimage each spring, summer and fall to the top of a mountain in a nearby State Park. On the way, my intention is to walk out of my worries into peace and to pray for whatever is in my heart. There are two ways to reach the top, a meandering carriage trail frequented by bikers and a path off the beaten track that traverses more secluded terrain. That is the one I always take.

The trail starts at the edge of a lake and goes down under evergreens along a path wet with dripping moisture from rocks. It comes out into the open, across rock slabs, down again under hemlocks into a cool area of reflected water. There I sit and listen to the flowing stream and meditate. Crossing to the other side over a fallen tree trunk, I ascend up a rocky path strewn with boulders. This eventually bursts out into the sunshine past low blueberry bushes before the last climb onto the ridge. From there, I look back down to the black and white speck that is my home, and out to the magnificent Catskill Mountains in the north. I have a sense of renewing an energy connection from my home to the Catskill Mountains and out to the universe and back again. Each time it's a new experience and I receive a different gift—a hawk overhead, a feather on the ground or a song in my heart.

Nancy Wood's two poems[4] below speak to the powerful nature of this mini-pilgrimage:

My help is in the mountain
 where I take myself to heal
 the earthly wounds
 that people give to me.

I find a rock with sun on it,
 and a stream where the water runs gentle,
 and the trees which one by one
 give me company.

So must I stay for a long time,
 until I have grown from the rock,
 and the stream is running through me,
 and I cannot tell myself from one tall tree.

Then I know that nothing touches me,
 nor makes me run away.
My help is in the mountain
 that I take away with me.

And...

Earth cure me. Earth receive my woe. Rock strengthen me. Rock receive my weakness. Rain wash my sadness away. Rain receive my doubt. Sun make sweet my song. Sun receive the anger from my heart.

Your Cancer Experience as a Healing Pilgrimage to Wholeness

One day during my cancer treatment I had an inspiring thought: "Aha, my cancer experience is itself a pilgrimage." I realized that the four traditional integral parts of a pilgrimage—the preparation, the journey itself, the arrival at my destination and returning full circle to home[5]—could all be applied to what I was going through. I envisioned myself as being on a path to health. With this perspective, my medical visits became sacred ports of call. As I took time to go inwards, I became more conscious of combining my inner and outer healing journeys. My medical visits were not in a separate world and the rest of my life in another. Realizing that everything is always inter-connecting brought a new spirit of openness to my healing process.

Preparing for your cancer journey

* Following a diagnosis, let your dreams and longing for healing inspire and guide you. Begin the preparation by deciding firmly to move towards healing. Carefully set your intention and then attend to the practical details of what's ahead. Preparation also includes choosing your personal and professional support teams, as well as doing research. These all enable you to make your medical visits with awareness.

Journeying

* Travel to your appointments—for tests, medical consultations with doctors and health care professionals. On the inner plane, picture the locations of your treatment as places that radiate significant healing energy, leading to a strong healing experience. It's best not to do this part of the journey alone. Have a companion with you at each visit and ask others to support you with their loving thoughts and prayers.

Arriving

* The next stage, arrival, happens when you have gone as far as you can or wish to on a particular treatment series or, say, a hospital stay. Pause to absorb what has happened thus far and offer thanks for the skill and kindnesses of those whom you have encountered. Ask for continued blessings.

How to apply the stages of a traditional pilgrimage to an experience of illness

Returning, integrating (and sharing its gifts, if you choose)

- As you return home to recuperate or re-group, take time for reflection and integration—give thanks, sort out which blessings or insights may be shared with friends and loved ones, and discover whether a different journey, perhaps a deeper one, now pulls you or whether you feel complete. Invite those who have been part of your healing journey to join with you in some way to mark the occasion, perhaps for a meal, a celebration or a healing circle...

4. Walk the Labyrinth's Ancient Path

A labyrinth is a sacred form or pattern laid out on the ground, used by many ancient cultures and spiritual traditions, including the Celts and indigenous Americans. Labyrinths are being re-created all over the place—inside and on the grounds of hospitals, parks and businesses as well as on church and private properties. A labyrinth provides the opportunity to center as we breathe, walk, meditate or pray.

There are two main types of labyrinths, one patterned after the one inside Chartres Cathedral[6] and the other patterned after those on the land of Ancient Crete. From ancient times there has been a strong connection between outdoor labyrinths and earth energies, bringing a timeless connection with nature and the feminine.[7]

I have walked a labyrinth for many reasons—healing, decision-making, peace of mind, reconnecting to my core and for help to go beyond hurried activities to essential truths and new depths of quiet. I can walk in the spirit of a pilgrimage. In fact I have contributed to this resurgence of labyrinths sprouting up all over the country, for there is now one in my front yard—open to those who wish to walk its curving paths.

What You May Experience Walking a Labyrinth

From the outer entrance, the labyrinth path weaves back and forth until you reach the center, balancing the right and left hemispheres of the brain and creating new neurological pathways. The path to the center is a metaphor for life. There are no wrong turns. It's not a maze with dead-ends to trick you. There are no unbreakable rules for walking a labyrinth. You may linger or stop for a while—the corners or turns are good places to do so. If you are walking with others, you may pass those ahead of you. Walking the labyrinth with others can be a powerful reminder that wherever you are on the path is just fine. Even if it appears that others are going in the opposite direction, all are traveling to the center at their own pace. Just as each day of your cancer experience may be different so too each time you walk will be different.

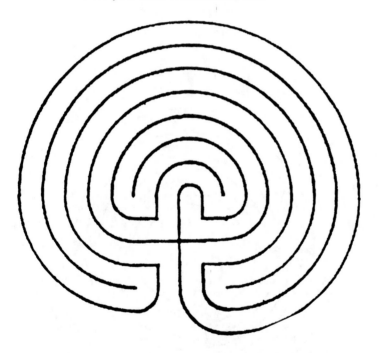

Labyrinth from ancient Crete

Painted portable canvas labyrinths can be set up anywhere on special occasions. It has also been found that tracing the lines of a labyrinth's pattern, following the path to the center with your index finger on a diagram, is an effective way to bring balance. Even if you are housebound, you can "walk" one in this way. Small wooden finger labyrinths are also available.

**If you wish
to follow a
labyrinth's
path**

- Do an Internet search, or ask around locally, to find a labyrinth near you.

- Choose an issue or a question for your walk: *At the entrance*, become aware of what you'd like to release—any anxiety or fears about your illness you may have been carrying.

- *As you walk inward*, think of yourself as walking into the very center of your being. Pray for healing and new strength. *In the center*, be still, feel the healing power of the earth beneath you feet and Divine energy all around you. Open your heart to blessing, insight and healing. *Walking out*, honor what you have awakened to with renewed trust.

- Look for announcements in your local newspapers of special events at a temporary labyrinth set up for the occasion. Group walks can be very powerful.

- Trace a labyrinth pattern with one of your fingers.

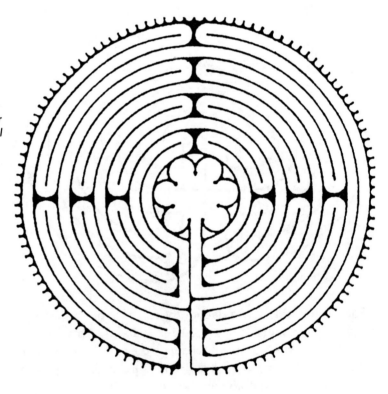

*Labyrinth on the floor
of Chartres Cathedral*

5. Ask for Help: Sacred Texts and Oracle Cards

People of all cultures have used signs and objects from nature to seek guidance when faced with suffering, confusion and challenge. Just as some people open a Bible, or another sacred text at random to ask for help, comfort and inspiration, others might choose a card with a symbolic picture on it to convey its message. All are based on the law of magnetic attraction. Since humans are both universal and individual, part of the great, undivided circle of Life, the passage or card you pick is personal and will resonate with what you need for the specific situation or concern. The cards offer a universal or spiritual perspective to personal experience.

There are many variations of cards. Traditional cards are available as well as a broad spectrum of modern boxed sets of cards and explanatory book taking inspiration from many sources such as angels, Goddesses, flowers and animals. I use meditation or oracle cards to give me insight into the issues surrounding a question in my heart. Times of rest between treatments and recuperation are especially opportune for receiving guidance. Once I chose the angel of "purpose" from the *Angel Card* deck. This little angel is steadily climbing a mountain with an ice-axe.[8] The card gave me encouragement to keep pursuing my goal for healing even when it felt like a slow uphill task at that time.

Puja Recently, feeling some anxiety about how this chapter would be received, I drew a card from the Motherpeace set.[9] It was the 9 of Swords. Nines are about completion. It shows one part of a personality cowering in terror and another part of the self rising up in strength and confidence, ready to confront the shadow. This heroic self can grab the fiery sword of liberation that is in front of her to cut through the confusion and fear of her own monsters. The message of the 9 of Swords was clear. I knew I had to express my own truths to finish the chapter.

You can use a card also to meditate upon and to set a theme or intention for the day. When I visited Findhorn, a spiritual center in Scotland, little angel cards were placed on the dining tables and on the doors to the kitchen to remind everyone of a quality to practice throughout that day. Each card was inscribed with one word such as grace, compassion, patience or joy, along with a delightful tiny picture of an angel illustrating the quality.

Consider asking for help from sacred texts or oracle cards

- Sit quietly—contemplate the day ahead or consider an issue for which you wish guidance.
- When you feel ready, intuitively choose a passage, a poem or a card at random.
- Stay open to receive the message contained in the words and/or picture, perhaps making some notes in your journal.

6. Ask for Help: Angels, Saints, Guides, Guardians and Non-Physical Beings

Most ancient and modern cultures accept the idea that we are not alone and that we can have contact with beings in other dimensions. Many people believe they can receive help for healing from these beings, for example, by calling on saints and angels in the west, protectors in the east, or spirit guides and animal totems in shamanic traditions. Christians and Jews might call on the archangel Raphael, whose name in Hebrew means "God Heals" or "God has cured." An internationally recognized children's research hospital known for its pioneering work in finding cures for children with cancer is named for St. Jude, patron saint of desperate causes. On the other hand, like the ancient Druids, indigenous Americans call on birds and animals as sacred guides and guardians for the qualities they represent such as eagle for spirit, hawk as messenger, bear for introspection and wolf as teacher.[10]

INTUITIVE AWARENESS

Although we all have psychic capabilities to communicate with other dimensions, our culture has not cultivated this natural ability. Children are often ridiculed for having "invisible playmates." As a result, their capacity for communicating with unseen beings gradually closes down. Other cultures do not limit children in this way and instead, have developed techniques to nurture intuitive awareness. People with such abilities are even revered as helpers and healers. If you have experienced glimpses of this phenomenon, it is not necessarily just your imagination. Asking for and receiving help from non-physical beings is just one of an infinite number of ways of connecting with universal truths.

Some people come to know their spiritual guides, helpers or angels in dreams or in meditation. They may not be able to prove their existence but they can feel a presence helping them. For example, Katie, one of the people to whom this book is dedicated, always invited a strong American Indian warrior, whom she had first met in her dreams, to be present during our energy work sessions. Spirit guides may take different forms according to your beliefs. Like angels, they are seen as God's messengers. Their job is to help you walk your path with confidence and to take you deeper into your own truth.

Some doctors and healers do pray for guidance and some even call on spirit guides to help them in their work. And of course, Edgar Cayce,[11] known as the 'Sleeping Prophet' is a well-known example of someone who went into self-induced trances and channeled medical advice for healing for over forty years. His transcribed words and remedies are still consulted today.

Others receive guidance out of the blue when they are least expecting it. Whether the guidance comes from the voice of a loved one who has passed away, from an "external" presence or from a hitherto-unknown part of themselves, the effect is startling.

Tory was not conciously asking for help, but she listened.

Tory One day, while driving, I heard a voice very clearly in my head say, "You know, you could have a recurrence." Since my initial diagnosis and lumpectomy eight years previously, I had been so certain that I was "cured" that I dismissed this as an unwelcome fear and forgot all about it. However, about a month later, again in my car, when I heard that voice in precisely the same conversational tone repeat the same phrase, it got my attention. After that, I found myself in odd moments idly stroking the site of my previous surgery. About six weeks later, I felt what was to be a sesame seed-sized lump. When my GP and surgeon both expressed strong doubt that this was anything to worry about, I insisted they *do a biopsy. They were both extremely surprised when the little "seed" turned out to be malignant—but I wasn't. The surgeon later praised me for "listening to my body." Whatever that voice was, I'm convinced it saved my life.*

Consider asking for help from unseen presences

- Remember back to when you were a child—did you have a favorite saint? A favorite relative who protected you when you were young, but who is no longer alive? A special kinship with a bird or animal?
- As an adult, have you felt a blessing presence in a dream?
- Call on whatever source feels intuitively healing for you.

An Abundance of Ways

Other ancient pathways to health, such as drumming circles, sweat lodges, vision quests and ceremonies, might be helpful to you. Perhaps you might choose to embrace the ancient ways of nature-based healing remedies and natural whole foods. If you are aware of the cycles of the moon, you might design healing rituals in alignment with its different phases. Like farmers of old, you may become more tuned into its influence to help you with activities that build strength as it waxes and or prune back as it wanes.

Tapping your inner spirituality and inviting the counsel of spiritual elders can also contribute to healing medical practices. More and more patients are seeking out such opportunities to supplement their modern protocols. Some doctors, patients and families feel it is time to explore ways of restoring the soul to medicine.

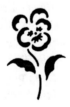

Moving Forward

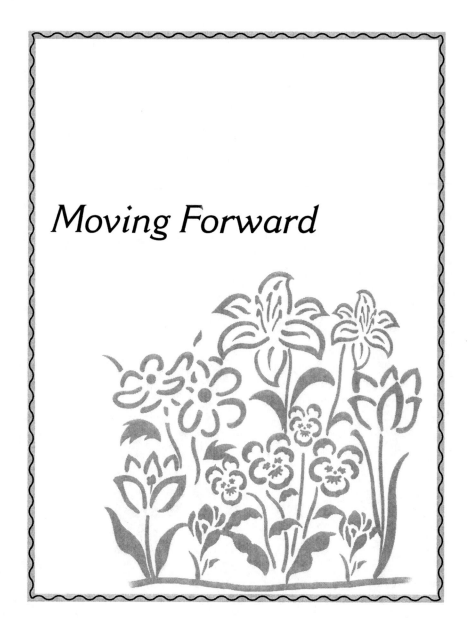

11

Towards the Best of All Possible Care

1. Past, Present, Future

THE CIRCLE

ONCE UPON A TIME LONG, LONG AGO, THE ARC, THE curve, the circle and spiral were central to the experience and expression of life. The circle, the simplest of all curves, has represented the cycles of life, day after night, season after season and generation after generation. It also represented eternity where, beyond time, there is no beginning and no end. Circles abound in nature—for example, concentric growth rings of a tree and ever-expanding circular ripples after a pebble has been thrown into still water. The circle was deeply woven into everyday life as people lived in round teepees, igloos or yurts, spent hours around the fire and worshipped in ancient circles of sacred stones.

In order to survive, a community or tribe depended on the cooperative effort of everyone, living in harmony with the seasons and the natural world around them. They came together in a circular chain of communication to make decisions for the good of all. This is still encoded in our genes. We have awareness of life cycles, and in our cancer experience, we can become sensitive to its treatment cycles.

THE LINE

As the ancient ways of the circle were displaced over the centuries by the conquering forces of aggression and power, a more important organizing symbol became the line. Its offspring were rectangles, squares, and boxes—shapes that became easily translated into multiple controllable units suitable for armies, factories and machines. For speed and efficiency, major highways cut right through the landscape; rectangular houses, office blocks and skyscrapers shot up. Taught in rows, we still queue up in lines, play sports on oblong fields and use repetitive machinery in gyms. Almost everywhere the direct line has supplanted the gentler curve.

A vertical hierarchical chain of command took over in institutions, and in most endeavors knowledge and research focused on increasingly intricate and specialized problems. Within medicine the development of very precise surgical skills, the mass production of medications and other advances benefited millions of people. But it came at a price. We began to grant institutional authority to those "above" us, according to the linear model. We lost our direct connection to nature and her abundant healing, herbal ways, and we unfortunately lost our appreciation of the whole web of life.

COMBINING THE GIFTS OF LINE AND CIRCLE

When we honor our longing for wholeness, connection, and cooperation, we can chart a way forward...

The challenge for our era is to find ways to unite the best of both the circle and the line, to reclaim that which has been lost, and integrate that which has been separated. Domination, fragmentation, and isolation will abound without this balance. When we honor our longing for wholeness, connection, and cooperation, we can chart a way forward to share the gifts of both, not only for ourselves, but for the good of our children and our children's children.

Nowhere is this new opportunity more evident than in the decisions we make about our bodies. Bodies are not just machines or things "to be fixed" by the doctor. They are very much alive with pulsating energy flowing through, constantly in flux and change.

Reclaiming Ancient Healing Practices

Physicians, practitioners and cancer patients are reclaiming that which has been lost or under-emphasized, by reintegrating the ancient ways of wholeness symbolized by the circle, and in medicine the wise serpent. For example Dr. Lewis Mehl-Madrona, inspired by his Cherokee grandmother, recognized how alienated his indigenous American patients felt in a modern hospital environment. When he included healing ceremonies and honored other traditional ways in his Western medicine practice, the beneficial effects were clear and recovery was more rapid.[1]

After all, as Black Elk, an Oglala Sioux Elder, taught, "You have noticed that everything that an Indian does is in a circle, and that is because the Power of the World always works in circles, and everything tries to be round... Everything the Power of the World does is done in a circle. The Sky is round, and I have heard that the earth is round like a ball, and so are all the stars. The wind, in its greatest power, whirls. Birds make their nest in circles, for theirs is the same religion as ours. The sun comes forth and goes down again in a circle. The moon does the same, and both are round. Even the seasons form a great circle in their changing, and always come back again to where they were. The life of a man is a circle from childhood to childhood, and so it is in everything where power moves"—including healing.

Dr. Christine Horner's book *Waking the Warrior Goddess*, with its program to protect against and fight breast cancer, tells how to harness the power of nature and natural medicines to achieve extraordinary health.[2] Dr. Horner awoke her own warrior Goddess to fight hard and long to get the Women's Health and Cancer Rights Act signed into law in 1998. In this book, she honors her debt to, and shares with us, the teachings of Ayurveda, an ancient system of healing from the East. As cancer patients learn more about the toxicity of our everyday environments, growing numbers are more eager to learn and integrate such positive, non-toxic ways to promote a healthier lifestyle.

DEVELOPMENTS IN INTEGRATIVE MEDICINE

Other physicians within the mainstream system are taking risks and making valiant efforts to bring about change. Many are willing to be more open, and offer a different kind of inclusive service in ways that will benefit us all. Dr. Andrew Weil, Dr. Bernie Siegel and Dr. Naomi Remen are among those who have become influential well-known advocates for a complementary and integrative approach. Newsletters such as the *Townsend Letter for Doctors and Patients* — (the "examiner of medical alternatives") include news of integrative protocols.

You can be sure that integrative health care is expanding when an increasing number of highly reputable medical institutions, such as Sloan-Kettering Cancer Center and Beth Israel Medical Center, are now offering integrative services such as acupuncture and other touch therapies, nutrition counseling, herbs and supplements as well as yoga and meditation classes. Duke Center for Integrative Medicine, linked to Duke University Medical Center in Durham, North Carolina, has a long commitment to integrative medicine. Its programs for cancer patients include Integrative Physician Consultations, Integrative Health Coaching, Acupuncture, Integrative Nutrition and Weight Management, Health Psychology, Movement and Fitness, and Bodywork. Other educational programs will be available to professionals and the public as well.

Until recently, many oncologists only had the opportunity to be trained in Western Medicine. This is changing and now, the training of physicians in the philosophy and practice of integrative medicine is welcomed by patients. The College of Medicine at the University of Arizona boasts the first university-based two-year fellowship in Integrative Medicine. Other institutions have a long track record of developing Integrative Medicine programs based on research.[3]

2. Good News and Hopeful Signs

EXCITING CHANGES AFOOT

We are in the midst of amazing developments in medicine, which, I believe, will take us beyond the boundaries of present thinking about the prevention and treatment of disease, including cancer. As research becomes widely disseminated via the Internet, our knowledge increases daily. Newly defined fields, for example DNA studies of cancer genes, fractal geometry, and minimally invasive techniques such as Radiofrequency ablation (RFA) or the Gamma knife and Cyberknife, represent useful directions for new therapies. Innovative investigations of consciousness reveal the extraordinary capacity of the mind to effect healing.[4] More and more studies document the importance of spirituality as an inner health resource. Some studies, as we have seen, show the positive effect of prayer and meditation,[5] while others reconnect us with the relevance of the worldview of ancient mystics, defying the boundaries of time, space and distance. Other new technologies, such as advanced biofeedback systems, originally developed for space exploration or war, are now thankfully being used for healing purposes. In the hands of a trained practitioner, the capacity of such systems to diagnose and treat vibrationally seems like science fiction.[6] We have an astonishing opportunity to be open to all the new possibilities for healing that abound.

We can forge holistic, inclusive partnerships with all of those willing to be team players. Some differences of opinion may actually help us define more clearly what is right for us.

It takes time, however, for new ideas to become widely accepted, and it's not always easy to be on the cutting edge of a shift in consciousness. As the saying goes, "Old habits die hard." It's often easier for us to abdicate power by looking up to the doctor as one who has the authority over *all* things medical and who can make decisions on our behalf, especially if family members advocate conventional solutions. Nonetheless, we must listen attentively to our inner sense of health and make some choices based on that, even if those who love us are not in total agreement. We can forge holistic, inclusive partnerships with all of those willing to be team players. Some differences of opinion may actually help us define more clearly what is right for us.

When Marion Woodman decided to receive complementary treatments for uterine cancer from a naturopath in addition to her mainstream treatments, her husband took exception and invited a close friend for fifty years, a medical doctor, to come for dinner. In the course of the conversation the doctor backed up his assertion that his wife should not do this. After their friend left, Marion quietly told her husband that she was going ahead with it. "He said, 'You can't do that.' 'I don't care,' I said. 'I will continue to go where my soul is recognized.' 'I understand that, Marion, but you can't split like that.' 'I'm not a bit split,' I said. 'Medical science can do its best for me and naturopathy can do its best. I'll take the best of both worlds.' "[7]

RECENT ADVANCES IN CANCER RESEARCH

I wrote the previous section in 2006, and since then, amazing developments have continued.

Cancer research has been expanding at an unprecedented rate. With improved technology and communications, research in one of the many types of cancer can be applied to other cancers very quickly.

With the personalized medicine revolution, as well as genomics research, physicians have the ability to analyze the genetic blueprint of a tumor and choose the most appropriate therapy for a patient's specific cancer.

Significant advances include the following:

- Radiation treatments can be specifically targeted—with a single dose of radiation delivered during surgery.
- Robotic surgeries are much less invasive, speeding up the recuperation process.
- Many chemotherapy drugs are much less toxic and therefore easier on the patient.
- Vaccines and viruses are used in new ways.[8] For example, who would have imagined using a modified polio virus to treat brain tumors or a herpes-based treatment for melanoma?
- Plant-based medicines, such as those derived from a rare plant found in the rainforest of Australia.[9]
- 3D mammography increases the accuracy of breast cancer diagnosis. If diagnosed, a patient may be advised to receive systemic therapy prior to surgery, for example, with anti-

estrogen therapy (which blocks the production or utilization of estrogen) or with monoclonal antibodies (mAbs or moAbs). These laboratory-produced molecules are engineered to attach to specific defects in cancer cells and fight them directly without harming healthy cells. Monoclonal antibody drugs are already available for a number of cancers, and clinical trials are under way studying their possible uses in nearly every type of cancer.

- Doctors can enlist a patient's own immune system with biological therapies, or immunotherapy, that use substances occurring naturally in the body to help fight a tumor.
- Older patients with blood cancers can now receive bone marrow/stem cell transplants. This was previously only available to those under thirty.
- 3D printing technology advances is another area to watch closely for artificial limb development for those who may have suffered an amputation due to cancer or other reasons.

Breakthrough V. False Hope?

One of the biggest challenges is to really understand cancer. Cancer continues to be elusive and keeps changing, attempting to be one step ahead of each new treatment. Often the media touts a possible new cure as a breakthrough when initial results of a Phase 1 trial are promising, even although numbers are very limited. Some new treatments do shrink tumors but very few live up to expectations in the subsequent phases of a trial, leading to possible disappointment.[10]

Cancer as a Chronic Disease

For many people, cancer is becoming a chronic disease. They are never free from the possibility of a recurrence even after a significant number of years, as in Ujjala's case (see pages 33, 34, 159). The third time around, Ujjala decided to accept a transplant (which she had not wanted to consider before).

Ujjala
Round 3: My Stem Cell Transplant

After 18 years of being in remission, my Lymphoma returned as a fast growing B cell. I needed a stem cell transplant. I had to start chemo again in November 2010. I had to be clear of the Lymphoma so I could proceed with the stem cell transplant. [11]

Every day I would draw a hot bath, light candles, and listen to a CD which helped me to imagine myself going through the transplant challenges successfully and I became more accepting of what was ahead.

There are two types of transplants, one in which you receive the cells of a donor (allogeneic), or one in which you receive your own cells, (autologous). I was to receive cells from a donor.[12] All I knew was that he was 27 years old and that we were a perfect match. I joked that he was the only perfect match I ever had—but I wasn't allowed to contact him for a full year!

I arrived at the center mid-January 2011. I was calm and centered, bringing with me items that I wanted to be surrounded by during my time in isolation—my lamp which gave my room a homey feeling, my purple blanket, and pictures of family and friends. Oh yes, my chicken hat…I would put it on at times when doctors or nurses came into the room—it was my comic relief. It worked. I would laugh and so would they!

Over the next three weeks, I had tubes in my chest and each arm. I was dealing with the ups and downs of the rigorous procedures before the transplant. On the days in isolation when I wasn't feeling weak, I would draw, watch nature documentaries, and keep my good sense of humor up with the doctors and nurses. I felt even more isolated when I went into A-Fib and was moved to a very tiny room. I wanted to run away and had to remind myself that this was temporary.

My transplant day finally came on February 1, 2011. I told the nurses and doctors that this was my wedding day—I was receiving cells from my perfect match, and they were my witnesses. They laughed and played along with me. It was anticlimactic after all I had gone through. The red blood entered my veins, and I was now AB positive instead of B positive. A whole new me was emerging—I was being reborn!

During the next twelve weeks, I stayed at Hope Lodge in New York City.[13] My sons arranged for different family members and friends to stay with me. It was such a humbling experience having so many different loved ones caring for me, making meals, going *shopping, and taking me to the hospital every day. My new outfit for many months to come was a mask and gloves.*

The downside of having a donor is that the transplant patient may experience a form of Graft vs. Host disease. I unfortunately have chronic GvsH, which can come back at any time, and I have had to deal with this throughout the last four years.

I thought, once I was home, I'd be on my way to total healing, but this wasn't true. I was on so many drugs that made me weak. As an energetic person, it was so hard to not be able to do anything. It was one thing to be in that state while in the hospital, but now, without a partner to help, it was much more difficult to accept.

A year after my transplant the hospital asked me if I wanted to hear from my donor—of course I said yes! I received a call from my "perfect match," Randy Wells, a Texas Navy man, stationed in San Diego. I was so excited to speak to him. He, my sons, and I have kept in touch. My sons surprised me by bringing Randy to NYC during the holidays two years ago. I cried; he cried, and we hugged and laughed. I couldn't stop thanking him for saving my life.

It has been a long journey back to health, but four years on, I'm pretty much back to being myself. I am so grateful that I am able to enjoy life because of the advances in stem cell transplants and those who become donors. I encourage people to become donors—it is as simple as taking a swab from the mouth that is put into a donor's registry.[14]

> *I am so grateful that I am able to enjoy life because of the advances in stem cell transplants and those who become donors.*

THE IMPORTANCE OF EARLY PREVENTION AND DETECTION

Of the 1.6 million new cancer patients in 2015 in the U.S., it is estimated that only 20-30% of the cancers are caused by direct genetic factors.[15] The rest are caused by environmental factors such as agricultural pesticides, tobacco, toxic toys, and an American diet—with excessive sugar and toxic additives—that has led to an obesity epidemic. In fact, cancers caused by obesity are actually expected to exceed tobacco-related cancers for the first time in recent history. This information is sobering. Individually and collectively, we are our own worst enemies if we tolerate and even condone behaviors that lead to cancer.

However, more people are realizing the need to hold the food and drink industries accountable to exclude or even minimize carcinogenic and other harmful ingredients. Taking personal responsibility, with a healthy diet, exercise, and sufficient sleep, will help prevent unnecessary diseases and cancers.

Cancer is no longer seen as one disease. It's a convenient umbrella for almost 40 diseases.[16] A correct early diagnosis is very important since treatment that is successful with one cancer may not work with another. There can be understandable circumstances that delay a correct early diagnosis. A doctor can misdiagnose a rare cancer, and unusual life circumstances can lead a patient to believe that factors other than cancer are causing physical and emotional symptoms. These two factors converged in Melissa's journey.

The value of friendship is vital when dealing with cancer. A supportive environment of friends can greatly enhance one's mood through the ups and downs of treatment. The encouragement and practical assistance of Melissa's friends is key in helping her cope with cancer.

Melissa
The Strength of Friendship

*The first time that I began to have strange symptoms, I attributed them to a trauma that had occurred at the high school where I taught— I had witnessed, and intervened in, a screwdriver stabbing. I did not seek medical assistance. I began crying frequently. I believed that the excessive crying was from Post Traumatic Stress Disorder. I sought out talk therapy and carried on. I attempted to have more fun, by playing music with my friends weekly. But I also began to misplace things, and my short term memory decreased dramatically. Still I did not seek medical help. When summer came, I started a tiling project in my bathroom and worked with my head down for a week, increasing the blood flow to my brain. I got some headaches, which I ASSUMED were the result of nighttime stressful teeth-grinding. I continued to self-medicate by increasing my dose of summer. I joined a drum circle and returned to regular Tuesday therapy sessions. I never missed a beat, **but I did miss the inner meaning of the headaches.***

I began to experience changes in speech. I was losing my ability to think of the words that I wanted to say, but that symptom was also disguised by my knowledge of vocabulary: I had little trouble finding replacement words to express myself. One day, I went to a friend's house to help her paint, and while taping off the floor, I grew nauseous and regurgitated my food. I believed this was caused by a week of working with chemicals. I fell asleep on the floor in an ad-

joining room. My friend arrived to find me there. She woke me and was startled that I was speaking in a garbled language; the aphasia made her think that I had possibly suffered a stroke. She insisted that I was rushed to a medical center an hour north of my home where I was misdiagnosed with a Glioma. The surgeon performed brain surgery the following day. When the extricated tissue was tested, it was revealed to be lymphoma, a rare brain cancer.

My mentor, Barbara, arranged for my transfer to a huge metropolitan cancer center. I started a chemotherapy regimen that quickly began to aid my improvement.

My friend Kate arrived at the hospital with delicious food and Netflix to help me through all of my weekend treatments. Her comfort and the time spent together laughing and enjoying one another meant the world to me and lifted my spirit. They dosed me with Chemo and shot me with targeted radiation, and I recovered.

I raced back to work, against advice from many, and did well for a little over a year before symptoms, such as a loss of short-term memory, began to return. Another good friend, Shamsi, decided that I needed to be checked out. When I went to the hospital, they discovered that another lymphoma had developed on the opposite side of my brain. This round of treatment was simpler in many ways. There was no surgery to recover from, and I understood the stages of medicine more thoroughly. My familiarity with the routine reduced my fear, and I received so much help thanks to a Google spread sheet created by Stephanie, a local acupuncturist. She encouraged Facebook friends to sign up to bring me meals, go for a walk with me, or just come and visit. This was wonderful since I wasn't allowed to drive while on Keppra. Without that signup sheet, my daily life would have been far more lonely, and my diet would not have been as varied and healthy. The kindness and generosity of friends has helped me through this challenging time. Shamsi, has moved in with me temporarily, and the comfort of companionship has aided greatly in defeating the blues as my treatment continues." [17]

THE COMING DIGITAL HEALTH REVOLUTION

For innovations that could totally change our future, we must look to technology which is transforming every aspect of our lives—including our health. The use of Smartphone apps and wearables (from companies such as Fitbit) is in its infancy, but powered by nanotechnology and cloud computing, it is growing and becoming increasingly sophisticated.

Apple, Microsoft, Samsung, and other major players are developing health devices using microelectromechanical systems (MEMS) sensors to enable measurements and feed the data into cloud-based platforms such as HealthKit. Wearing a MEMS device linked to a personal Smartphone, individuals will have the capability to monitor and re-direct their health according to feedback they can read on their screen. Action can be taken BEFORE a health crisis like a heart attack or a cancer diagnosis occurs. With 24/7 monitoring, a result of artificial intelligence systems, individuals will be given recommendations about solutions, such as medications needed.

However the digital health revolution is not without risk. Just as tobacco companies hid the carcinogenic effects of smoking, there is a likelihood that there is not open disclosure about the possible health risks of wearing digital devices. Already there is recognition that cell phones worn constantly next to a specific body part and other extensive use of wireless technology can trigger changes in health.[18]

Our Voices and Actions are Making a Difference

Although many issues affecting our health appear to be beyond our control, it is possible, by our individual actions and by joining with others, to influence change in cancer's health policy issues. We can become informed and speak up concerning the health issues we care about. We can create a groundswell from below to combat the trickle-down effect of policies made from above by people whose agendas seem to be other than health.[19]

First of all we can bring about change by aligning ourselves with the "**precautionary principle**." This idea affirms that if the consequences of an action are unknown, but are judged to have some potential for major or irreversible *negative* consequences, then it is better to avoid that action. The concept includes risk prevention, cost effectiveness, ethical responsibility towards maintaining the integrity of natural systems, and the fallibility of human understanding.[20] The precautionary principle guides us, for example, to become aware of the link between our health and the environment. As we learn to "do no harm" in the choices we make by reading labels and becoming informed consumers and advocates for our own health, we are contributing to the common good. We can refuse to buy products that have been unleashed on the market without adequate testing as to their safety and the harm they might cause. At the same time we can follow a good diet, exercise, and take time to reduce our stress levels, all of which are now known to contribute to health without harm.

Here are examples of issues where the voices and actions of cancer survivors and those who care about quality of health care are already awakening awareness and building support.

It is now recognized that towards the end of treatment, a review and post-treatment "survivorship" recommendations must be offered and discussed. Without such care, cancer survivors are needlessly at greater risk both of recurrence and of developing new tumors. What can we do? The National Coalition for Cancer Survivorship (NCCS) recommends that we:

- Request a formal consultation with our doctors at the end of treatment in order to be provided with a cancer care summary (of diagnosis and treatment) and a survivorship care plan (for follow-up care after primary cancer treatment).[21]

- Become educated about local resources to help cancer survivors deal with emotional and practical issues, such as discrimination in the work place or inadequate access to health insurance.

- Network with others to highlight this issue by, for example, joining the NCCS's Cancer Advocacy Now™ group.[22]

The movement challenging people to change the system ethically by being selective about what their money supports is growing.[23] The criteria for healthy, **socially responsible investing** with regard to health include 1) Avoid causing illness, disease and death and 2) Avoid destroying or damaging the environment. If you are in the fortunate position of having investments or money put away for retirement in IRAs or ROTHs, it may no longer make sense to invest savings in businesses that manufacture known cancer pollutants while at the same time you are recovering from the very serious effects they may have had on your health.

It is now recognized that towards the end of treatment, a review and post-treatment "survivorship" recommendations must be offered and discussed.

A similar situation exists with regard to **socially responsible cancer fundraising**. Some companies ask for your money to support cancer research, while manufacturing consumer products containing toxic chemicals implicated as risk factors for cancer. For example, cosmetic and personal care items contain parabens and phthalates,[24] both of which are endocrine disrupters. *"Think Before You Pink"* is spearheading a movement calling for people to ask, and be selective about, where their cancer donations are going.[25] The need is for more money to be directed to research into environmental pollutants and toxic chemicals, which to date remains vastly under-funded.

There are, of course, other important issues that you might choose to focus on.[26] As we—patients, families and practitioners—continue to dialog and make our voices heard on a range of issues affecting our health, we are capable of bringing positive change to our healthcare system in general and cancer care in particular. We are all in this together.

PEACE, LOVE AND COURAGE

"Cancer can be the teacher of truth… Such illness opens the doors to one's own heart, and between heaven and earth."[27] These words rang true to me. None of us knows exactly what the turning seasons of life will bring, but we can be sure that the only certainty is change. I hope this book, in its many aspects, helps and encourages you as you move from diagnosis towards healing.

Now I leave you with the words of an ancient Egyptian prayer for those setting out on a pilgrimage, "Be safe and well. **Peace, love and courage.**"[28]

Puja *My experience with cancer, when using ancient healing practices as well as modern medicine, was more than a physical experience. It was a heart-centered path towards greater trust and deeper truths, with many little miracles along the way.*

Endnotes

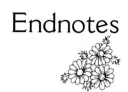

CHAPTER 2

1 HealthAlliance Hospital Oncology Support Program in Kingston, NY, go to www. hahv.org. Breast Cancer Options offers excellent weekly research updates and vitamin discounts. www.breastcanceroptions.org

CHAPTER 3

1 See *Appendix 2*, Section 5: Consulting, Treatment Information and Referral Services

2 I also like the *Cochrane* CAM definition as it attempts to be applicable to any nation or culture: "Complementary and alternative medicine (CAM) is a broad domain of healing resources that encompasses all health systems, modalities, and practices and their accompanying theories and beliefs, other than those intrinsic to the politically dominant health system of a particular society or culture in a given historical period. CAM includes all such practices and ideas self-defined by their users as preventing or treating illness or promoting health and well-being. Boundaries within CAM and between the CAM domain and that of the dominant system are not always sharp or fixed." Cochrane Collaboration: www.cochrane.org

3 Thermography, using FDA-approved infra-red camera equipment, can detect the increased metabolic heat associated with the increased vascularity of most suspicious growths, sensing the "thermal signal" or "hot spots" of pathology often years in advance of a mass detected by X-Ray. Thermography is a physiologic test, and mammography is a test of anatomy. Both tests provide their own unique information and *when both are used*, a better picture of health or disease can be seen.

To be accurate, thermography *must* be used only in the hands of trained personnel, using the correct type of cameras under controlled conditions (uniformly cool temperature etc.) It can be a valuable tool as an adjunctive exam to provide a more comprehensive picture of ongoing breast health. Several studies show that monthly self-exam, annual physician check-up, yearly thermography and mammography, where indicated, increase the effectiveness of early detection to greater than 95%. In a recent FDA approved study (USC Norris Cancer Center, Parisky, MD et al.) published in the January 2003 issue of the American Journal of Radiology (AJR), thermal imaging was shown to have a 97% sensitivity for normal breast tissue in patients who had mammograms identifying the breast to have a tumor or calcification requiring a biopsy. Thermography however is not 100% accurate. For further info, go to www.breastthermography.org

4 "QXCI" (Quantum Xrroid Consciousness Interface) On the one hand, from a mechanistic perspective, it was amazing to me that my practitioner's computer would register information which she could then use when we were miles apart; yet from an energy perspective it was quite understandable.

5 Physicians, who are also trained in Anthroposophy (the teachings of Rudolph Steiner)—more common in Europe—often recommend the self-injection of iscador (mistletoe) for cancer prevention.

6 As of 2015, there are 141 accredited medical schools in the United States which grant M.D. degrees, and 30 grant D.O. (Doctor of Osteopathy) degrees. 110 teach CAM courses within the regular training of doctors. Over twenty offer post-graduate CAM courses for practicing doctors.

7 Barrie R. Cassileth, PhD, Chief, Integrative Medicine Service, Memorial Sloan Kettering Cancer Center in NYC states, "We know from extrapolation of previous research that about 8-10% of newly diagnosed patients—tissue biopsy-diagnosed patients with all kinds of cancers—go directly to an alternative practitioner. This is a very serious problem. It's a small percentage of the total, but that small percentage turns out to be a very large number of human beings that we have to worry about. These are patients who will go to an alternative practitioner for six months or a year while their disease continues to grow unabated. When they realize that it's not working, they eventually go back to the hospital where they were diagnosed or to some other hospital or cancer center. Usually they are beyond hope of cure and sometimes beyond hope of treatment at that point. It's a very, very sad situation."

CHAPTER 6

1 You may wish to create tabs for other practitioners not mentioned thus far. The examples below are not exhaustive and are in no way to be interpreted as specifically validating modalities included or judging any modalities omitted.

Mainstream: Radiation Oncologist; Radiologist; Specialists e.g. for second opinions; Plastic Surgeon; Other.

Complementary or alternative (CAM): Acupuncturist; Ayurvedic MD; Chiropractor; Energy Healer (such as Polarity; Reiki; Therapeutic Touch; etc); Herbalist; Homeopath; Massage Therapist; Medical Intuitive; Naturopath; Practitioners in Bach Flower Essences, Biofeedback, Cranial Sacral Work, Essential Oils, Shiatsu; Other.

Other professionals: Aesthetician; Cosmetician; Dream Facilitator; Hair/wig Consultant; Health Kinesiologist; Hypnotherapist; Life Coach; (Medical) Social Worker; Personal Trainer; Prosthesis Maker, Psychotherapists—especially body-centered psychotherapies such as Bio-energetics; EFT; Rubenfeld Synergy; Spiritual Practitioners such as Minister/Rabbi/Priest/Imam; Psychic; Spiritual Counselor; Yoga Teacher; Other.

2 Other Reports/Results might include Biofeedback; Biopsy; Bone Marrow test; CA21; CTscan; Chemotherapy; Genetic Information; Mammography; Medication; MRI; Pap Smear; Pathology; PET Scan; Pulse; Second Opinion; Scope; Sonogram; Surgery; Thermography; Ultrasound; X-Ray; Other.

3 According to a detailed article in *Consumer Reports* March 2006 on *The New Threat to Your Medical Privacy*, "Under the provisions of the Health Insurance Portability and Accountability Act (HIPAA), healthcare providers have the right to share your data for several purposes: to treat you, which means, for example, they may discuss your case and send data about you to a radiologist about which ankle to X-ray; to process your insurance claim; and to respond to requests from public-health authorities, law enforcement, and your employer if you were hurt at work." That's

the positive side. However, "HIPAA also allows healthcare providers to share information with healthcare business associates. So notes from your psychotherapy session may be given to your insurers' employees for "training purposes," and your demographic information and the dates that you received treatment might be used for fund-raiser activities supported by your hospital or doctor's office.

4 For information, go Disability Rights section of the Department of Justice's website. www.justice.gov/crt/about/drs/

Taking time off to accommodate a disability would be through the Family and Medical Leave Act (FMLA). However, reasonable accommodation would be provided under the Americans with Disabilities Act (ADA)…

Reasonable Accommodation and The Americans With Disabilities Act (ADA): Reasonable Accommodation should be established by putting your request in • writing to your supervisor. Be clear about your request. Put down your disability or diagnosis and treatment schedule. For example you might say: "I am currently receiving treatment for cancer which qualifies me as a person with a disability under the Americans with Disabilities Act (ADA). As a qualified person with a disability, I am formally requesting 'reasonable accommodation' under the ADA. In particular, I am requesting modification of my work schedule to accommodate my need for treatment over the next ten weeks. As I will be receiving treatment every Tuesday and Thursday from 3:00 p.m. until 5:00 p.m., I am requesting that I be able to make up these four hours by working one and a quarter additional hours on Monday, Wednesday and Friday." Remember, under 'reasonable accommodation', and as an employee who qualifies for reasonable accommodation, you are still required to perform the 'essential functions' of the position for which you were hired. However, if you were no longer able to lift heavy objects but this is not a significant or essential function, it could be transferred to another employee. The best way to achieve an effective reasonable accommodation is to put your request in writing and set up a meeting with your supervisor to discuss the possibilities. You should also know that it is unlawful to discriminate against a person because they are perceived to have a disability. For example: if an employer thinks someone has a particular disability and discriminates on that basis, this would be a violation of the ADA. For more information about the ADA, reasonable accommodation and other employment provisions of the ADA contact a local Independent Living Center or ADA Technical Assistance Center.
    –provided by Douglas Hovey, Executive Director, Independent Living Inc.

5 www.estateplanning.com

6 When preparing your Living Will and your Healthcare Proxy, "FIVE WISHES," available from www.agingwithdignity.org, is a useful resource. 1-888-5-WISHES / 1-888-594-7437. The Five Wishes are for: "1. The person I want to make care decisions for me when I can't; 2. The kind of medical treatment I want or don't want; 3. How comfortable I want to be; 4. How I want people to treat me; and 5. What I want my loved ones to know."

The American Bar Association has a comprehensive online toolkit: www.abanet.org/aging/toolkit/home.html

7 www.personallegacyadvisors.com or www.personalhistorians.org

CHAPTER 7

1 Benson MD, Herbert. *The Relaxation Response.*

2 Robert Monroe started The Monroe Institute in Virginia. www.monroeinstitute.org

3 *Health Journeys* provides a wide range of image specific audios for illness created by BelleRuth Naparstek, www.healthjourneys.com 1-800-800-8661

4 As a result of research, Blue Cross-Blue Shield of California offers to provide a guided imagery audio to patients undergoing surgery. By paying for a $17 audio they save an average of $2,000 per surgery in shorter hospital stays. (*The New Medicine* broadcast on PBS, April '06)

5 Simonton MD, O. Carl, Stephanie Matthews-Simonton and James Creighton. *Getting Well Again.*

6 At the Menninger Foundation.

7 Porter, Garrett and Patricia A. Norris PhD. *Why Me? Harnessing the Healing Power of the Human Spirit* contains Garrett's script and drawings with Dr. Norris's perspective.

8 Garrett was helped by meeting Dr. Jerry Jampolsky, founder of The Center for Attitudinal Healing and by reading *There is a Rainbow Behind Every Dark Cloud* written by children at that center. www.ahinternational.org

9 Woodman PhD, Marion. *Bone: Dying into Life*, page 27. Dr. Woodman is a Jungian analyst, author, and leader in the field of feminine psychology.

10 E.g. *Health Journeys'* audio, *General Wellness*; (See 3 above); Ticia Agri's *The Ribbon Breath Meditation* www.meditationhealing.com

11 The Centerpointe Research Institute introduced me to *Holosync®* technology. www.centerpointe.com.

12 *Alive Inside* is an uplifting exploration of the effect of music on the mind and the brain—DVD. Also check out www.colorsinmotion.com/touchstone.html

13 Yosaif August of Healing Environments International, Inc, has developed bedside curtains with a serene view of a mountain stream or a tropical beach and accompanying audio to promote healing. www.bedscapes.com

14 Hunt PhD, Valerie. *Infinite Mind: The Science of Human Vibrations*, page 48.

15 Unfortunately manufacturers are not required to list phthalates.

16 Barrie Cassileth, PhD, (Chief, Integrative Medicine Service, Memorial Sloan Kettering Cancer Center) states, "One of the effective complementary modalities is massage. We have certainly found that to be the case at Memorial…. There is definitely a measured physiologic effect…. We've actually learned that foot massage for bed-ridden patients helps them get out of bed and walk more quickly and more easily."

17 Cassileth B.R. and A.J. Vickers. Integrative Medicine Service, Memorial Sloan Kettering Cancer Center, New York. *Massage Therapy for Symptom Control: Outcome Study at a Major Cancer Center.*
"Massage is increasingly applied to relieve symptoms in patients with cancer. This practice is supported by evidence from small randomized trials. No study has examined massage therapy outcome in a large group of patients. At Memorial Sloan Kettering Cancer Center, patients report symptom severity pre- and post-massage therapy using 0-10 rating scales of *pain, fatigue, stress/anxiety, nausea, depression and*

'*other.*' Changes in symptom scores and the modifying effects of patient status (in or outpatient) and type of massage were analyzed. Over a three-year period, 1,290 patients were treated. Symptom scores were reduced by approximately 50%, even for patients reporting high baseline scores. Outpatients improved about 10% more than inpatients. Benefits persisted, with outpatients experiencing no return toward baseline scores throughout the duration of 48-hour follow-up. These data indicate that massage therapy is associated with substantive improvement in cancer patients' symptom scores." PMID: 15336336 [PubMed—indexed for MEDLINE].

18 SmartBells classes for cancer patients and survivors work well. SmartBells inventor, Paul Widerman, plans to make a new movement and wellness product, HEART, available soon.

19 Quoted in Mayer, Jerry and John P. Holms. *Bite-size Einstein.*

20 I believe that Thomas Berry, author of *Dream of the Earth,* was right when I heard him say at an International Transpersonal Association conference in Ireland that "we Westerners no longer live in a 'universe.' Indigenous peoples live in a universe with the stars, stones, trees, creeks, and the four directions. Until we recover the universe, *our greater self,* we'll never recover from an alienation that shrivels the soul..."

21 Cousins, Norman. *The Anatomy of an Illness.*

22 Frankl, Victor. *Logotherapy—Man's Search for Meaning.*

23 LeShan, Lawrence. *Cancer as a Turning Point* and other books.

24 Shivani Goodman's audio programs are available at www.youheal.com

25 Bays, Brandon. *The Journey.*

CHAPTER 8

1 Dr. Winifred Rushforth OBE, one of the first women doctors to graduate in Edinburgh, Scotland in 1908, who became an important mentor to me late in her life, introduced me to the "four h's".

2 Dr. Bach noticed that there was a correlation between the types of intestinal toxemia and what he called the "mentals" of a patient, and he later went on to pioneer a form of vibrational medicine, the Bach Flower Essences, as he sought non-invasive forms of treatment. www.bachcentre.com

3 Arising out of their own experience, Louise Hay and others have popularized the art of attributing likely emotional and mental causes to illnesses. This can be very helpful although there is a definite danger in the oversimplification of a cookbook approach to body symbolism.

4 Chopra MD, Deepak. *Ageless Body Timeless Mind: The Quantum Alternative to Growing Old.*

5 The Center for Consciousness Studies at the University of Arizona is leader in this field. www.consciousness.arizona.edu

6 Emoto, Masaru. *The Hidden Messages in Water.*

7 Dr. Elisabeth Kübler-Ross, author of *Death and Dying,* first identified these stages in her work with terminally ill patients. Later it became clear that these feelings could be present in any situation of loss.

8 LeShan, Lawrence. *Cancer as a Turning Point,* and other excellent books on cancer.

9 Dossey MD, Larry. *Healing Words: The Power of Prayer and the Practice of Medicine*.

10 For more about perceptions of God, see Chapter 9.

11 From Marion Woodman's intensely personal journal of her cancer experience, *Bone: Dying into Life*.

12 Progoff, Ira. *At a Journal Workshop*. This basic text for using the *Intensive Journal* includes many ways of having an inner dialog.

CHAPTER 9

1 Dr. Irene Goodall's experience of cancer was woven throughout *"One Man's Journey,"* paralleling Robert Perkins' journey through the Canadian wilderness on Channel 13 WNET New York, 1/23/05.

2 Ecclesiastes 3:6

3 Osho: *Osho Transformation Tarot*, page 115.

4 "Sacred Secrets, Cellular Mysteries." Article by Sondra Barrett PhD in *EarthLight*, Winter 2005. www.mysticmolecules.com

5 John of God comes to Omega Institute, Rhinebeck, NY, from time to time. eOmega.org

6 www.rosalynlbruyere.org includes a calendar of training courses led by Rosalyn L. Bruyere.

7 E.g. The Consciousness Research and Training Project holds seminars in meditation and healing authorized by Lawrence Le Shan. www.CRTP.org

8 Brown, Norman O. *Love's Body*.

9 Bruyere, Rosalyn L. *Wheels of Light: Chakras, Auras and the Healing Energy of the Body*. Chapter 10 includes a discussion of cancer and its treatment from an energy perspective.

CHAPTER 10

1 For example, Commonweal is a nonprofit health and environmental research institute in Bolinas, California. www.commonweal.org. The Commonweal Cancer Help Program is a week-long residential support program for people with cancer.

2 This synthetic estrogen, once used in attempts to treat women at risk for miscarriage, was later discontinued after it was found to lead to various cancers.

3 Thomson, Puja A. J. Article originally in *Creations* magazine on "Pilgrimage—Deepening Your Relationships Through Travel." www.rootsnwings.com

4 From *Spirit Walker* by Nancy Wood, drawings by Frank Howell; and from *Hollering Sun*. For more of my favorite Nancy Wood poems, see *Many Winters—Prose and Poetry of the Pueblos*.

5 Cousineau, Phil. *The Art of Pilgrimage—The Seeker's Guide to Making Travel Sacred*.

6 Atress, Lauren. *Walking a Sacred Path—Rediscovering the Labyrinth as a Sacred Tool*.

7 Curry, Helen. *The Way of the Labyrinth—A Powerful Meditation for Everyday Life*.

8 *Angel Cards*, part of *The Transformation Game*, designed by Kathy Tyler on the Findhorn community, are available in bookstores or online.

9 Noble, Vicki. *Motherpeace* cards and book.

10 Sams, Jamie and David Carson. *Medicine Cards—the Discovery of Power Through the Way of Animals.*

Andrews, Ted. *Animal-Speak* (includes a dictionary of animal, bird, and reptile symbolism.)

11 Association for Research and Enlightenment, Inc. 800-333-4499
www.edgarcayce.org

CHAPTER 11

1 Mehl-Madrona MD, Lewis. *Coyote Medicine.*

2 Horner MD, FACS, Christine. *Waking the Warrior Goddess.*

3 For example, Osher Center for Integrative Medicine at University of California, San Francisco. www.osher.ucsf.edu/about-us/
University of Texas at Austin Integrated Health Program for students associated with the Mental Health Center of the university. http://www.cmhc.utexas.edu/index.html

Holistic Health Program at Western Michigan University. www.wmich.edu/holistic

4 The Center for Consciousness Studies at the University of Arizona, is the epicenter for new research in this field, encouraging the promotion of open, scientifically rigorous and sustained discussions of all phenomena related to the mind. www.consciousness.arizona.edu/

5 Dossey MD, Larry. *Healing Words.*

6 An example of this is QXCI (see also Chapter 3, endnote 4).

7 Woodman, Marion. *Bone: Dying Into Life.*

8 "A vaccine enlists the patient's own immune system in the fight against disease— engineering key immune cells in ways that essentially turn them into tiny tumor-fighting 'ninja warriors.'" (AARP Bulletin, Dec. 2014)

Also CBS *60 Minutes* Report by Scott Pelley followed brain cancer patients in a Duke University clinical trial of a therapy that uses a re-engineered polio virus to kill cancer cells on 3/29/15.

9 There has also been much excitement over what experts are calling a "cancer-curing" drug. Researchers were able to extract a chemical from a rare plant found in Australia that has the ability to eat cancerous cells and completely remove them in a few days. Clinical trials have been recently approved for the drug known as EBC-46. This drug is being viewed as an alternative for those whose chemotherapy has not worked or whose bodies may be too fragile for it.

10 There are more than a half-dozen companies with genetically engineered viruses making their way through the development path: www.forbes.com/sites/arlene-weintraub/2015/03/30/heres-what-60-minutes-didnt-tell-you-about-the-miracle-glioblastoma-treatment/

11 Memorial Sloan Kettering Cancer Center is one of 41 National Cancer Institute-designated Comprehensive Cancer Centers, with state-of-the-art science flourishing side by side with clinical studies and treatment.

12 The Bone Marrow Foundation www.bonemarrow.org helps families and patients. 1-800-365-1336. Most hospitals will make this information available and find a donor for patients.

13 One of the lodges run by The American Cancer Society at 132 West 32nd St. NYC, N.Y. 10001 (800-227-2345 www.cancer.org/hopelodgenyc.) It provides housing to people from other states as well as from foreign countries. Ujjala highly recommends Hope Lodge. It's free for cancer patients and caretakers and is a beautiful place to spend time while healing during treatment. The social workers at many hospitals can arrange housing for a patient as long as a caretaker can stay with the patient.

14 The National Marrow Donor Program, 1-888-999-6743, is entrusted to operate the Be The Match Registry. It is the largest, most diverse marrow registry in the world. www.bethematch.org 1-800-627-7692

15 Charlie Rose interviewed CEO Robert W. Stone and 2 medical researchers of the City of Hope on cancer research and new treatments for cancer on Channel 13 2/25/15 11PM. This program was an exceedingly clear overview and informed much of the new writing in this chapter.
www.cityofhope.org/comprehensive-cancer-center

City of Hope has a history of excellence in biomedical research, patient-centered medical care, and community outreach.

16 Ibid

17 In September 2015, Melissa completed her autologous stem cell transplant at Sloan Kettering with stem cells harvested from her own blood. She is now at home for a 3 – 12 month gradual recuperation period. Friends continue to offer essential varied support.

18 In May 2015, 190 scientists from around the world appealed to the United Nations, The World Health Organization and the United States to take action to protect humans and animals from Wireless Technology.
www.businesswire.com/news/home/20150511005200/en/International-Scientists-#.Vh1TGbyVPeg
Since this appeared on the BusinessWire (A Berkshire Hathaway company), it indicates that it is being taken seriously in the business world too.

Also www.bioinitiative.org

19 Financial and political institutions all too often appear to have tremendous power to override compassionate factors. Medicine has become big business and the effects of corporate greed can impinge on health care. Drug companies occasionally skew research, corporate-sponsored lobbyists influence the regulation of environmental toxicity, and non-medical personnel make decisions regarding the payment of insurance benefits, all to our detriment and their profit. We can help shift the balance.

20 Since 1998, SEHN, The Science and Environmental Health Network, has been the leading proponent in the United States of the Precautionary Principle as a new basis for environmental and public health policy. SEHN engages communities and governments in the effective application of science to protect and restore public and ecosystem health at local and state levels. www.sehn.org

21 Go to *My Survivorship Wellness Plan, Part 7* of *My Hope & Focus Cancer Organizer* by Puja A. J. Thomson for clear guidelines to help you create such a plan with your doctor.

22 www.canceradvocacy.org A project of the National Coalition for Cancer Survivorship.

23 www.ethicalinvesting.com

24 You may not have heard of phlalates, as manufacturers are not required to list them. For a list go to www.breastcanceroptions.org

25 www.thinkbeforeyoupink.org   A project of Breast Cancer Action.

26 Health issues that may become significantly more important are
  • electro-pollution, due to studies linking cell phone use to the increase of cancer, especially in children and young persons, as yet denied by the cell-phone industry
  • possible legislation to limit freedom of choice regarding vitamins and health care (Codex Alimentarius)

  • hydrofracking

  • lack of labeling of genetically engineered (GMO) foods

27 From a personal reading from Emmanuel channeled by Pat Rodegast, Sept. 2004.

28 Cousineau, Phil. *The Art of Pilgrimage.*

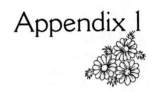

Build Your Own
Yellow Pages

All Your Cancer-Related Contacts
& Frequently Used Resources—at Your Fingertips!

Your personal *Yellow Pages* may be comprised of the following 13 sections or "pages." (You might need more than one sheet of paper for some of them. The pages to follow are templates for setting them up.)

1. Frequently-used Telephone/Email Contacts
   & Emergency Numbers
2. Chronological Cancer Log
3. Personal Contacts
4. Mainstream Medical Health Professionals
5. Complementary Health Professionals
6. Labs and Other Facilities Giving Reports
7. Pharmacies & Medications; Vitamins, Minerals & Supplements
8. Health Insurance, Legal & Financial Contacts
9. Possible Leads
10. Favorite or Most-frequently-used Resources
11. How Others Can Help
12. Thank You List
13. Where to Find It

Keeping these pages up-to-date not only benefits you: some pages will also give you a ready reference for your family and friends—even for your doctor. For example, make sure your support team members each have a copy of the contact information for your professional team, and your health providers have a copy of the page with your personal emergency contact numbers.

PAGE 1. Frequently Used Telephone/Email Contacts

Place this list wherever it is most accessible.

Name	Telephone	Email

Emergency Contact Numbers

Add your emergency telephone contact numbers below and add your primary ICE (In Case of Emergency) numbers to your cell phone contact list.

Primary contact_____

If unavailable, contact _____

Next of kin _____

Friend _____

Walk-In Medical Clinic _____

Hospital Emergency Room _____

Ambulance, Police, Fire _____

If in doubt, call 911.

EMERGENCY MEDICAL DATA

Medical conditions_____

Allergies _____

Medications _____ Blood group _____

Dr.'s name and tel #_____

PAGE 2. CHRONOLOGICAL CANCER LOG

Create an overview of your cancer history for yourself and others. You will be able to give a copy to all your health care providers when they request such information.

Name _____ age _____ date of birth _____

Address _____

Home phone _____ work phone _____

Blood type _____ Social Security # _____

Next of kin/person to contact in emergency _____

Allergies (with medications, if any) _____

Previous surgeries, if any, with dates _____

Other medical conditions and medications _____

Take as much space as you need to build an accurate record.
Note the date each time you add new information.

a. **First noticeable symptoms, if any, when?** _____

   Pre-treatment visits, prior to your current diagnosis, if any, when? _____

b. **First cancer diagnosis and date** _____

   Given by _____

   Location _____

   Notes (such as doctor's follow-up recommendations and your feelings) _____

c. **Other consultations, tests and results *prior to* your treatment decision:**

   Health Professional _____ date _____

   Facility _____

   Purpose _____

   Findings/recommendations _____

d. **My initial treatment decision** _____ date _____

   1st Treatment date _____ location _____

e. **Follow-up treatments:** _____

Add all consultations, tests and test results, adjuvant therapies, chemotherapy drugs, and prescribed medications in chronological order under the heading below:

With _____ or under the supervision of _____

Purpose _____

Notes _____

Use extra pages as you go along

PAGE 3. Personal Contacts

	Name	Address	Telephone	Email
Close family members, if any				
Personal support team				
Other friends & personal contacts				
Centers, support groups, organizations				

PAGE 4. MAINSTREAM MEDICAL HEALTH PROFESSIONALS

Include your mainstream doctors, nurses, specialists, oncology support contacts etc. *Asterisk those who have a copy of your living will and health care proxy. For each, list:

Professional's name _____

Specialty _____

Office address _____

Tel, fax & email _____

Name of office _____

Receptionist, if any _____

Secretary, if any _____

Nurse, if any _____

Best way to contact office _____

Hospital affiliation _____

Your patient # _____

PAGE 5. COMPLEMENTARY HEALTH PROFESSIONALS

Include all your complementary care doctors, nurses, acupuncturists, naturopaths, healers, massage therapists, chiropractors, cranial-sacral body-workers and others. *Asterisk those who have a copy of your living will and health care proxy. For each, list:

Professional's name _____

Modality _____

Office address _____

Tel, fax & email _____

Name of office _____

Receptionist, if any _____

Secretary, if any _____

Nurse, if any _____

Best way to contact office _____

Hospital affiliation _____

Your patient #, if any _____

PAGE 6. Labs and Other Facilities Giving Reports

For each, list:

Name of facility _____

Contact person _____

Address _____

Tel/fax _____

Email _____

Best way to contact _____

PAGE 7. Pharmacies & Medications

Pharmacy _____

Contact person _____

Address _____

Tel/fax _____

Email _____

Best way to contact _____

For each medication note the following information.

Name of medication _____ generic or brand? _____

Prescribed by _____ date _____

For _____ dosage _____

Date began _____ instructions _____

Doctors informed of new prescription _____

Positive/negative results/side effects _____

Vitamins, Minerals & Supplements

For each vitamin, mineral or supplement, note the following information.

Name _____

For _____ dosage _____

Start date _____ (special) instructions _____

Doctors/practitioners informed of supplement _____

Positive/negative results/side effects _____

PAGE 8. HEALTH INSURANCE, LEGAL & FINANCIAL CONTACTS

* Asterisk those who have a copy of your will, your living will and healthcare proxy.

Primary Health Insurance Company _____

Membership ID _____ effective date _____

Plan name_____ policy or group number _____

Contact person, if any _____

Tel/fax/email _____

Secondary Insurance Company _____

Membership ID _____ effective date _____

Plan name_____ policy or group number _____

Contact person, if any _____

Tel/fax/email _____

Lawyer _____

Office address _____

Tel/fax/email _____

Office receptionist, if any _____

Financial Advisor_____

Office address _____

Tel/fax/ email _____

Consultant and/or tax preparer_____

Office receptionist, if any _____

PAGE 9. Possible Leads

List each person or organization you've heard about, and might like to contact at some point.

Name _____

Address (if known) _____

Tel/email/website (if known) _____

Reason for contacting _____

Source of information _____

PAGE 10. Your Favorite/Most Frequently Used Resources

If you use a computer for record keeping, note where this information is stored.

Articles

Books

National organizations

Websites

Other—such as medical search organizations

PAGE 11. How Others Can Help

Create a list of tasks you would appreciate others doing. Keep it handy —in your date book or beside your phone—for those times when people ask how they can help.

Help needed	Suggested to/offered by	Time frame

PAGE 12. Thank You List

Here you can keep a record of any gifts of love, or kind thoughtful actions, no matter how small; and when and how you have expressed your gratitude.

Person to thank	For	Thanked by call/card/email	Date

PAGE 13: Where to Find It

For ease of mind, list where you keep all your important information. Provide a copy for your legal representative and close family members.

Item	Bank safety deposit box	Home firebox	Filing cabinet	Lawyer's Office	Wallet	Other:
Located in						
Computer Passwords						
Back-up drive						
Financial						
Bank accounts						
Credit cards						
IOUs						
IRAs/Roths						
Investments						
Retirement and pension						
House / home						
Deed / Mortgage						
Rental						
Insurance						
Car (+title & registration)						
Health						
House						
Other						
Legal						
Health care proxy						
Living will						
Organ donor info.						
Power of attorney						
Will/Trust						
Personal						
Birth certificate						
Divorce/separation papers						
Driver's license						
Funeral arrangements						
Marriage certificate						
Passport						
Taxes						
Social Security #						
Other						

Appendix 2

Directory of Resources

1. **Organizations & Websites**
2. **Newsletters & Magazines**
3. **Books**
4. **Audios & Videos**
5. **Consulting, Treatment Information & Referral Services**
6. **Miscellaneous Resources**

Please note: I have not personally reviewed all these resources, which have been suggested by many patients and practitioners. *MEDLINEplus* offers helpful guidelines for evaluating websites and healthy web surfing: www.nlm.nih.gov/medlineplus/evaluatinghealthinformation.html *and* www.nlm.nih.gov/medlineplus/healthywebsurfing.html. Please re-read Section 5 of Chapter 6, especially "About using the internet" and its cautions. Most resources apply to cancer in general, not to a specific cancer.

1. Organizations & Websites

Free online resources for information about conventional medicine as well as complementary, alternative and integrative treatments.

Acupuncture. www.medicalacupuncture.org and www.acupuncture.com
American Academy of Environmental Medicine. www.aaemonline.org/ 1-316-684-5500

American Cancer Society. www.cancer.org 800-227-2345
Helps locate cancer-related resources in your area and offers interactive assistance with conventional treatment decisions. Includes a link to a survivors' network; local cancer groups; transport to appointments, leaflets on aspects of cancer, including social; and books for children.

American Society of Clinical Oncology (ASCO). www.asco.org 571-483-1300

Annie Appleseed Project. www.annieappleseedproject.org
Information, education and advocacy for people with cancer seeking complementary, alternative (CAM) and 'natural' approaches. 561-749-0084

Association of Cancer Online Resources. www.ACOR.org 212-226-5525. Home to a large network of online support groups, with a searchable archive. Joining a list requires a password, available at no cost, to protect participants' privacy.

www.bolenreport.com Provides insight into the Western Health care system.

Cancer Care, Inc. www.cancercare.org 1-800-813-HOPE (4673) Excellent free tele-conferences and support.

Cancer Monthly. www.cancermonthly.com Information about cancer treatments.

Cancer Support Community www.cancersupportcommunity.org Complementary and Alternative Medicine section contains "recent news" to keep members up-to-date.

Cancer Treatment Centers, Hospitals and Universites with informative websites about cancer including the following:

Cancer Treatment Centers of America. www.cancercenter.com 800-931-0599 800-615-3055

Duke University. www.dukehealth.org/Services/IntegrativeMedicine/ index

Mayo Clinic. www.mayoclinic.org A broad range of topics — causes, symptoms and treatments for 30 types of cancer.

MD Anderson Cancer Center at the University of Texas. www.mdanderson.org

Memorial Sloan Kettering Cancer Center. www.mskcc.org includes an excellent link to herbs and their interaction with chemotherapy.

Schachter Center for Complementary Medicine. www.schachtercenter.com for extensive complementary information.

University of Arizona Program in Integrative Medicine. www.integrativemedicine.arizona.edu

University of Maryland Center for Integrative Medicine. www.compmed.umm.edu

Caregiver Action Network. www.caregiveraction.org
1130 Connecticut Ave NW, Suite 300, Washington, DC 20036 202-454-3970

www.caringbridge.org Create a free website to connect with family/ friends during treatment.

www.castleconnolly.com Peer-reviewed top doctor guides.

Center for Advancement in Cancer Education. www.beatcancer.org

Center for Medical Consumers. www.medicalconsumers.org Excellent archive of past advocacy updates.

Childhood and Adolescent Cancer Support

> **American Childhood Cancer Organization (ACCO).** www.acco. org 855-858-2226. Peer support, advocacy and information including organizations for financial assistance.

> **www.kidshealth.org** For parents, teens and children.

> **Kids Konnected.** www.kidskonnected.org 949-582-5443. Support network for children with family members with cancer.

> **Young Survival Coalition.** www.youngsurvival.org

Clinical Trials. www.ClinicalTrials.gov A database linking patients to medical research (more than 9,000 clinical trials that address cancer and other diseases). Search by condition or location or call the National Cancer Institute (NCI) at 800-4-CANCER.

Commonweal. www.commonweal.org PO Box 316, Bolinas CA 94924 415-868-0970 Director: Dr. Rachel Remen. Help for physicians, nurses and medical students; retreats for cancer patients.

> Linked to **Institute for the Study of Health & Illness (ISHI)** Director: Dr. Michael Lerner. Not-for-profit health and environment research institute. ISHI healer's art curriculum is offered at many medical schools. www.ishiprograms.org

www.drweilsplan.com Andrew Weil, MD.

www.HappyChemo.com has a useful financial support resource guide, offering freebies and discounts.

Healthfinder. www.healthfinder.gov Reliable health information, hand-picked from government agencies, nonprofit organizations, and universities (US Dept. of Health and Human Services site).

Homeopathy.
National Center for Homeopathy. www.homeopathic.org

Hospice and Palliative Care.
Caring Connections. www.caringinfo.org

International College of Integrative Medicine. www.icimed.com 419-358-0273

www.latestagecancer.com

www.lotsahelpinghands.com

Medical Thermography International. www.medthermonline.com

MediCope Mapping Project. www.medicope.com Helpful hints for breast cancer patients.

MEDLINEplus. www.nlm.nih.gov/medlineplus/ Information on treatments, support groups, national foundations, clinical trials and medical literature, under the National Cancer Institute (NCI); a link to PubMed, a service of the National Library of Medicine (NLM) that provides access to more than 12 million references. www.nlm.nih.gov/medlineplus/directories.html

National Cancer Institute. www.cancer.gov & **Cancer Information Service** 800-422-6237 Research and statistics plus personal responses to questions about cancer from specialists at regional centers throughout the U.S. Personal online help through the "LiveHelp" link, and a useful selection of brochures.

National Center for Complementary and Alternative Medicine. www.nccam.nih.gov

National Coalition for Cancer Survivorship. www.canceradvocacy.org 1010 Wayne Avenue, Suite 315, Silver Spring, MD 20910 301-650-8868. General Info 877-622-7937. See Section 5 for excellent free audio kit: *The Cancer Survival Toolbox®*.

National Health Freedom Coalition. www.nationalhealthfreedom.org Working towards freedom of access to healing and to the health care of your choice.

Naturopathy. For registered naturopathic doctors www.naturopathic.org For association of oncology naturopaths www.oncanp.org

Nutrition:

Food and Nutrition Information Center. fnic.nal.usda.gov

Organic food. www.wilson.edu/robyn-van-en-center Information on community supported agriculture; also www.organicconsumers.org

HerbMed. www.herbmed.org

Hippocrates Health Institute. www.hippocratesinst.org Raw live foods, detoxification and cleansing.

www.integrativenutrition.com

Palliative Care. www.getpalliativecare.org

Patient Advocate Foundation (PAF). www.patientadvocate.org 800-532-5274. Non-profit organization serving as an active liaison between the patient and insurer, employer and/or creditors to resolve insurance, work and financial matters as a result of cancer.

Pharmaceutical and Research Manufacturers of America (PhRMA). www.phrma.org Keeps updated directory of Prescription Drug Patient Assistance Programs.

Pregnant with Cancer Network. www.hopefortwo.org

University of Arizona Center for Consciousness Studies. www.consciousness.arizona.edu At the forefront of new research, encouraging the promotion of open, scientifically rigorous, sustained discussions of all phenomena related to the mind.

2. Newsletters & Magazines

Celebrate Life! The Newsletter of the Oncology Support Program at HealthAlliance of the Hudson Valley, 105 Mary's Avenue, Kingston, NY 12401. 845-338-2500 x4453
www.hahv.org/service/celebrate-life-newsletter Free

Cure Magazine. Cancer updates, research & education www.curetoday.com Offers free subscriptions.

Julian Whitaker. www.drwhitaker.com *Health & Healing: Your Definitive Guide to Alternative Health and Anti-Aging Medicine;* Plus 8 books and a booklet: *"What Would I do if I had Cancer"* 1-888-349-0484

The Moss Reports. www.cancerdecisions.com Ralph Moss has written many books on the cancer industry and alternative treatments. PO Box 1076, Lemont, PA 16851. 800-980-1234. Free online newsletter.

Townsend Letter. *The Examiner of Alternative Medicine.* For doctors and patients. www.townsendletter.com
911 Tyler Street, Port Townsend, WA 98368-6541. 360-385-6021.

Life Extension Magazine. Life Extension Foundation www.lef.org
800-678-8989

Living and Working with Cancer Workbook—a resource for working women created by Cosmetic Executive Women Foundation (supported by *Roche)* www.cancerandcareers.org

3. Books

Books about Cancer, Healing & Treatment

For books about specific types of cancer, please ask your doctor or check the Internet.

Alschuler ND, FABNO, Lise N. & Karolyn A. Gazella. *The Definitive Guide to Cancer, 3rd Edition: An Integrative Approach to Prevention, Treatment, and Healing.* 2010.

Alschuler ND, FABNO, Lise N. & Karolyn A. Gazella. *The Definitive Guide to Thriving After Cancer.* 2013.

Anderson, Greg. *Cancer: 50 Essential Things to Do.* Revised 2013.

Andron PhD, Michael & Ben Andron. *The Essential Guide to Energy Healing.* 2012.

August, Yosaif & Bernie Siegel, MD. *Help Me to Heal.* 2004.

Bach MD, E. & F.J. Wheeler, MD. *The Bach Flower Remedies.* 1998.

Balch & Balch. *A Prescription for Nutritional Healing. Fifth edition.* 2010.

Benson MD, Herbert. *The Relaxation Response.* 2000.

Bloch, Annette & Richard. *Fighting Cancer.* 2008.

Borysenko PhD, Joan. *Mending the Body, Mending the Mind.* Updated and Revised, 2009.

Brennan, Barbara Ann. *Hands of Light*. 1988.

Bruyere, Rosalyn L. *Wheels of Light: Chakras, Auras and the Healing Energy of the Body*. 1994.

Campbell PhD, T. Colin. *Whole: Rethinking the Science of Nutrition*. 2013.

Canfield, Jack, Mark Victor Hansen & David Tabatsky. *Chicken Soup for the Soul: The Cancer Book*. 2009.

Carlson PhD RPsych, Linda E. & Michael Speca PsyD RPsych. *Mindfulness-based Cancer Recovery: A Step-by-Step MBSR Approach to Help You Cope with Treatment and Reclaim Your Life*. 2012.

Chopra MD, Deepak. *Ageless Body Timeless Mind, The Quantum Alternative to Growing Old*. 1994.

Chopra MD, Deepak. *Quantum Healing*. 1990.

Clegg, Holly and Gerald Miletello MD. *Eating Well Through Cancer*. 2006.

Coleman MD, C. Norman. *Understanding Cancer*. 2006.

Cousins, Norman. *The Anatomy of an Illness as Perceived by the Patient*. 2005.

Dossey MD, Larry. *Healing Words: The Power of Prayer and the Practice of Medicine*. 1995.

Dossey MD, Larry. *The Extraordinary Healing Power of Ordinary Things: 14 Natural Steps to Health and Happiness*. 2007.

Eden, Donna & David Feinstein. *Energy Medicine: Balancing Your Body's Energies for Optimal Health, Joy, and Vitality*. 2008.

Elias, Jason. *Feminine Healing*. 1997.

Epstein MD, Samuel. *Cancer-Gate: How to Win the Losing Cancer War.* 2005

Fein, Ellen. *Not Just a Patient: How to Have a Life When You Have a Life-Threatening Illness*. 2006.

Gawande MD, Atul. *Being Mortal: Medicine and What Matters in the End*. 2014.

Gawler, Ian. *You Can Conquer Cancer*. 2015.

Gerber MD, Richard. *Vibrational Medicine*. 2001.

Gordon, Jim. *Comprehensive Cancer Care*. 2001.

Groopman, MD, Jerome. *How Doctors Think*. 2008.

Halpern, Susan. *The Etiquette of Illness: What to Say When You Can't Find the Words*. 2004.

Halvorsen-Boyd, Glenna & Lisa K. Hunter. *Dancing in Limbo: Making Sense of Life after Cancer*. 1995.

Hay, Louise. *You Can Heal Your Life*. 1984.

Heymann, Jody. *Equal Partners: A Physician's Call for a New Spirit of Medicine*. 2000.

Horner MD, Christine. *Waking the Warrior Goddess*. 2007.

Jenkinson, Stephen. *Die Wise: A Manifesto for Sanity and Soul*. 2015.

Kübler-Ross, Dr. Elisabeth. *On Death and Dying.* 2014.

Le Shan, Lawrence. *Cancer as a Turning Point.* 1994.

Lerner, Michael. *Choices in Healing: Integrating the Best of Conventional and Complementary Approaches to Cancer.* 1996.

Lipman MD, Frank & Danielle Claro. *The New Health Rules: Simple Changes to Achieve Whole-Body Wellness.* 2015.

Lorig, Kate, et. al. *Living a Healthy Life with Chronic Conditions.* 2012.

Mehl-Madrona MD, Lewis. *Coyote Medicine.* 1998.

Morra, M. & E. Potts. *Choices: The Most Complete Sourcebook for Cancer Information.* 2003.

Motz, Julie. *Hands of Life.* 2000.

Moyers, Bill. *Healing and The Mind.* 1995.

Myss, Caroline. *Why People Don't Heal and How They Can.* 1998.

National Institutes of Health, National Cancer Institute. *Eating Hints: Before, During, and After Cancer Treatment.* 2012.

Northrup MD, Christiane. *Mother-Daughter Wisdom.* 2006.

Northrup MD, Christiane. *The Wisdom of Menopause (Revised edition).* 2012.

Northrup MD, Christiane. *Women's Body, Women's Wisdom.* Revised 2010.

Northrup MD, Christiane. *Goddesses Never Age.* 2015.

Price ND, Lisa A. and Susan Gins MA, MS, CN. *Cooking through Cancer Treatment to Recovery.* 2015.

Prinster, Tari. *Yoga for Cancer 2014.* www.y4c.com

Quillin, Patrick. *Beating Cancer With Nutrition.* Revised 2005.

Remen MD, Rachel Naomi. *Kitchen Table Wisdom—Stories That Heal.* 2006.

Reynolds-Price, Anthony. *A Whole New Life: An Illness and a Healing.* 2003.

Rossman MD, Martin L. *Fighting Cancer From Within: How to Use the Power of Your Mind.* 2003.

Rossman MD, Martin L. *Guided Imagery for Self-Healing.* 2000.

Schwartz, Anna L. *Cancer Fitness — Exercise Programs for Patients and Survivors.* 2004.

Servan-Screiber MD PhD Rev., David. *Anticancer.* 2009.

Sherman MD, Janette D. *Life's Delicate Balance.* 2000.

Siegel MD, Bernie. *Love, Medicine and Miracles.* 1990.

Silver, Maya & Marc Silver. *My Parent Has Cancer and It Really Sucks.* 2013.

Simonton, O. Carl, Stephanie Matthews-Simonton & James Creighton. *Getting Well Again.* 1992.

Steingraber, Sandra. *Living Downstream: An Ecologist's Personal Investigation of Cancer and the Environment.* 2010.

Steinman, D. & S. Epstein. *The Safe Shopper's Bible.* 1995.

Stearn, Jess. *Edgar Cayce: The Sleeping Prophet.* 1989.

Thomson, Puja A. J. *My Hope & Focus Cancer Organizer*. 2013.

Walters, Richard. *Options: The Alternative Cancer Therapy Book*. 1992.

Woodman, Marion. *Bone: Dying Into Life: A Journal of Wisdom, Strength and Healing*. 2001.

Miscellaneous Books (about Meditation, etc)

Andrews, Ted. *Animal-Speak*. 2002.

Atress, Lauren. *Walking a Sacred Path: Rediscovering the Labyrinth as a Sacred Tool*. 2006.

Bays, Brandon. *The Journey*. 2012.

Berry, Thomas. *Dream of the Earth*. 2006.

Borysenko PhD, Joan. *Women's Journey to God*. 2001.

Brach, Tara. *Radical Acceptance: Embracing Your Life With the Heart of a Buddha*. 2004.

Brown, Norman O. *Love's Body*. 1990.

Cousineau, Phil. *The Art of Pilgrimage: The Seeker's Guide to Making Travel Sacred*. 2000.

Curry, Helen. *The Way of the Labyrinth: A Powerful Meditation for Everyday Life*

Dispenza, Dr. Joe. *Breaking the Habit of Being Yourself: How to Lose Your Mind and Create a New One*. 2013.

Dyer, Wayne. *Power of Intention*. 2010.

Emoto, Masaru. *The Hidden Messages in Water*. 2005.

Frankl, Victor. *Man's Search for Meaning*. 2006.

Goleman, Daniel. *The Meditative Mind*. 1996.

Hanh, Thich Nhat. *The Energy of Prayer: How to Deepen Your Spiritual Practice*. 2006.

Hunt PhD, Valerie. *Infinite Mind: The Science of Human Vibrations*. 1996.

Kabat-Zinn, Jon. *Full Catastrophe Living: Using the Wisdom of the Mind to Heal the Body*. 1990.

Kabat-Zinn, Jon. *Wherever You Go, There You Are*. 2005.

Le Shan, Lawrence. *How to Meditate*. 2005.

Livingston, Kathryn E. *Yin, Yang, Yogini*. 2014.

Mipham, Sakyong. *Ruling Your World*. 2006.

Newberg MD, Andrew & Mark Waldman. *How God Changes Your Brain*. 2010.

Noble, Vicki. *Motherpeace*. 1994.

Osho. *The Silence of the Heart: Talks on Sufi Stories (The Perfect Master, Volume 2)*. 2009.

Osho. *Meditation: The First and Last Freedom*. 2004.

Osho. *The Silence of the Heart: Talks on Sufi Stories (The Perfect Master, Volume 2)*. 1992.

Progoff, Ira. *At a Journal Workshop.* 1992.

Roshi, Suzuki. *Zen Mind, Beginner's Mind.* 2011.

Rozien MD, Michael F. & Mehmet Oz MD. *YOU: The Owner's Manual, (Updated and Expanded).* 2008.

Rude, Paul. *Making Miracles.* 2011.

Sams, Jamie & David Carson. *Medicine Cards: Discovery of Power Through the Way of Animals.* 1999.

Schultz PhD, Mona Lisa. *Awakening Intuition: Using Your Mind-Body Network for Insight and Healing.* 1999.

Seligman EP PhD, Martin. *Authentic Happiness: Using the New Positive Psychology to Realize Your Potential for Lasting Fulfillment.* 2004.

Thomson, Puja A.J. *My Health & Wellness Organizer.* 2013.

Tolle, Eckhart. *A New Earth.* 2008.

Tolle, Eckhart. *The Power of Now.* 2004.

Thondup, Tulku. *Boundless Healing: Meditation Exercises to Enlighten the Mind and Heal the Body.* 2001.

Travis MD MPH, John W. & Regina S. Ryan. *The Wellness Workbook: How to Achieve Enduring Health and Vitality.* 2004.

Vaughn, Francis. *Awakening Intuition.* 1979.

Weed, Susun. *Herbal Wise.* 2003.

If your local library doesn't have a book, request it through the inter-library system.

4. Audios & Videos

The Cancer Survival Toolbox® Building Skills That Work For You available as a set of CDs or online, in English and Spanish and Chinese (print only). 1-877-866-5748 www.canceradvocacy.org An excellent FREE resource from the National Coalition for Cancer Survivorship.

www.cancercenter.com/community/discussions/blog/

www.ihadcancer.com/h3-blog

www.well.blogs.nytimes.com/category/body/cancer/

www.positivepause.com Visual images for meditation.

American Cancer Society: Audios www.cancer.org 800-227-2345

Bruyere, Rev. Rosalyn L. *Chakra Healing* (CD). www.rosalynlbruyere.org/bookstore.html

Dossey MD, Larry. *One Mind* (CD). 2013.

Dossey MD, Larry. *The Power of Prayer.* Amazon Audible Audio Edition 2014.

Eden, Donna. *The Energy Medicine Kit.* Healing. Includes DVD and CD

Goodman, Shivani. Audio programs from www.youheal.com

Healing Journeys. www.healingjourneys.org Offers conference videos and DVDs:

Health Journeys. www.healthjourneys.com by Belleruth Naparstek. CDs and DVDs. Podcasts and videos: Excellent guided imagery and affirmation healing audios such as General Wellness, Cancer, Chemotherapy, Radiation, Surgery and other specific illnesses. 1-800-800-8661

Hepburn, Elizabeth. *Better & Better Series.* DVDs and CDs. Healing programs for pre- and post-surgery patients and their caregivers. www.elizabethhepburn.com

MD Anderson Center. Videos of patient conversations. See page 206.

Monroe, Robert. www.monroeinstitute.org *Hemi-Sync* CDs and DVDs

Moyers, Bill. *Healing and the Mind.* PBS Video series.

Osho. Meditation CDs such as *Osho Nadabrahma* (Music by Deuter) or *Osho Chakra Sounds* www.osho.com

Robin DC CCN, Carol. *Transforming Cancer Surgery* and other guided meditations. 1-800-657-8119 www.imagerymeditation.com

The New Medicine. DVD. www.thenewmedicine.org

Thomson, Puja A.J. *ROOTS & WINGS—for strength and freedom*, a CD of guided imagery and meditations to transform your life, with music by Richard Shulman and a companion workbook. www.rootsnwings.com

5. Consulting, Treatment Information and Referral Services

American Medical Association. www.ama-assn.org Official directory of medical specialists. To check out physicians in the US, click on "doctor finder."

The Moss Reports. www.cancerdecisions.com Phone consulations for cancer patients.

CANHELP. www.canhelp.com 800-364-2341. Cancer treatment information and referral service.

6. Miscellaneous Resources

RETREATS

Cancer as a Turning Point, From Surviving to Thriving. ™ Weekend conferences with speakers, performers, music, humor, healing stories, and networking time. www.healingjourneys.org FREE

The Stowe Weekend of Hope. www.stowehope.com Annual conference for cancer survivors and their families. FREE

Commonweal Retreats. See section 1.

Smith Center for Healing and the Arts. www.smithcenter.org Offers cancer programs and retreats.

OTHER

Advance Directives
    American Bar Association. www.abanet.org/aging/toolkit/
    www.agingwithdignity.org *Five Wishes*, comprehensive living will and
    health agent forms. 888-594-7437.

Belief Net. www.beliefnet.com offers daily meditations online.

Carr, Kris. *Crazy Sexy Cancer.* Paperback, movie, blog.

www.cleaningforareason.org Free house cleaning for four months for
    women who are in treatment, with note from MD. *Cleaning for a Reason*
    will make arrangements with a participating maid service.

Corporate Angel Network. www.CorpAngelNetwork.org 914-328-
    1313. Arranges free travel for cancer patients to and from treatment in the
    unused seats of corporate aircraft flying on routine business.

Electromagnetic fields and health BioInitiative Report:
    www.bioinitiative.org

www.estateplanning.com

www.ethicalinvesting.com

Ethical will. www.personalhistorians.org (Association of personal
    historians) or www.yourethicalwill.com Personal legacy advisaors.

Healing Environments International, Inc. www.bedscapes.com
    Bedside curtains with a serene view, with audio, to promote healing.

Nursing Drug Handbook thepoint.lww.com/ndh2015 (if necessary, enter a
    later year).

Science & Environmental Health Network. www.sehn.org Promotes
    the Precautionary Principle.

Silent Unity. www.unity.org/prayer 24-hour prayer hotline: U.S.
    800-NOW-PRAY (800-669-7729), international 01-816-969-2000.

www.thinkbeforeyoupink.org

www.saunex.com For state-of-the-art far infrared portable sauna.

Index

Please check the *Directory of Resources* for websites, organizations, books, and other cancer resources.

Order copies of our award-winning book

At your local bookstore, or

Call: 845-255-2278 and pay with your Visa or MC

E-mail: orders@rootsnwings.com. Include name, address, phone, quantity and preferred method of payment.

Online: http://www.rootsnwings.com/aftershock and click on *Add to Cart* button.

Mail: Roots & Wings Publishing, PO Box 1081, New Paltz, NY 12561

Indicate number of book(s) @ $19.95 per book

Add US shipping & handling: $5.75 first book, plus $1.50 each additional book.

NY state residents, please add 8% sales tax.

Other works by Puja Thomson:

Roots & Wings for Strength and Freedom—
Guided Imagery and Meditations to Transform Your Life CD
ISBN 978-1-928663-08-9

Roots & Wings Workbook—
Guided Imagery and Meditations to Transform Your Life
Revised Edition   ISBN 978-1-928663-06-5

Roots & Wings Workbook & CD   Revised Edition   ISBN 978-1-928663-07-2

My Hope & Focus Cancer Organizer—Manage Your Health and Ease Your Mind
Revised edition   ISBN 978-1-928663-11-9

My Health & Wellness Organizer —
An Easy Guide To Manage Your Healthcare—And Your Medical Records
ISBN 978-1-928663-12-6

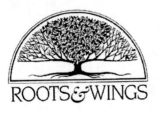

For more information:
www.rootsnwings.com/aftershock

ROOTS *&* WINGS
PO Box 1081, New Paltz NY 12561

puja@rootsnwings.com

CPSIA information can be obtained
at www.ICGtesting.com
Printed in the USA
FFOW02n2210280216
21802FF